PREPPER'S NATURAL MEDICINE

Lifesaving Herbs, Essential Oils and Natural Remedies for When There Is No Doctor

Cat Ellis

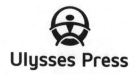

Ulysses Press

Copyright © 2015 Cat Ellis. Design and concept © 2015 Ulysses Press and its licensors. All rights reserved. Any unauthorized duplication in whole or in part or dissemination of this edition by any means (including but not limited to photocopying, electronic devices, digital versions, and the Internet) will be prosecuted to the fullest extent of the law.

Published in the U.S. by
ULYSSES PRESS
P.O. Box 3440
Berkeley, CA 94703
www.ulyssespress.com

ISBN: 978-1-61243-438-4
Library of Congress Control Number 2014952014

Printed in Canada by Marquis Book Printing

10 9 8 7 6 5 4 3 2 1

Acquisitions Editor: Kelly Reed
Managing Editor: Claire Chun
Project Editor: Casie Vogel
Editor: Susan Lang
Proofreader: Lauren Harrison
Indexer: Jay Kreider, J S Editorial
Front cover and interior design: what!design @ whatweb.com
Cover artwork: © images72/shutterstock.com
Layout: Jake Flaherty

Distributed by Publishers Group West

NOTE TO READERS: This book has been written and published strictly for informational and educational purposes only. It is not intended to serve as medical advice or to be any form of medical treatment. You should always consult your physician before altering or changing any aspect of your medical treatment and/or undertaking a diet regimen. Do not stop or change any prescription medications without the guidance and advice of your physician. Any use of the information in this book is made on the reader's good judgment after consulting with his or her physician and is the reader's sole responsibility. This book is not intended to diagnose or treat any medical condition and is not a substitute for a physician.

This book is independently authored and published and no sponsorship or endorsement of this book by, and no affiliation with, any trademarked brands or other products mentioned within is claimed or suggested. All trademarks that appear in ingredient lists and elsewhere in this book belong to their respective owners and are used here for informational purposes only. The authors and publishers encourage readers to patronize the quality brands mentioned in this book.

This book is dedicated to my best friend, soul mate, and loving husband, Eddie. Thank you for your love, patience, and humor. You are my hero, now and always.

CONTENTS

CHAPTER 1

INTRODUCTION

Have you ever wondered what you would do if there were no pharmacy? What if access to health care were suddenly cut off? Are you concerned about the rise of drug-resistant bacteria? Do you have a backup plan? *Prepper's Natural Medicine* can help you put your plan in place.

Natural medicine is everywhere, even growing up through the cracks of sidewalks and occupying vacant lots. The addition of a medicinal herb garden at home and some simple stored items can provide you and your family with a wealth of effective remedies as well as valuable barter items in the event our current systems fail.

This guidebook teaches the basics of crafting natural medicines, gives detailed information on the therapeutic properties of 50 different herbs (plus a few extras), and shares some time-tested remedies for emergencies, first aid, and common complaints. Everything you need to learn how to make your own formulas for your specific needs is in this book. I've also provided a list of books, suppliers, and other resources for your further study.

As an herbalist who is also a prepper, I am concerned about antibiotic resistance, emerging viruses, and the risks posed by chronic disease. I am concerned that the United States currently ranks #60 in maternal mortality in spite of (or because of) the many interventions now considered part of normal birth in our hospitals. I am concerned about the Centers for Disease Control and Prevention (CDC) reports that one of every two adults in the United States has a chronic illness. I am concerned about the political shenanigans over health coverage and the suppression of natural medicine and nutrient-dense foods by our government's regulatory agencies in favor of corporate food. I am also concerned that we are moving to a system in which access to health care and type of treatment are determined by our government rather than health care professionals.

I wrote this book to help others get ready for a number of scenarios. During a crisis, pharmacies and hospitals will be among the first places raided. Millions of people on maintenance drugs will suddenly be without medicines that their bodies depend on for normal functioning. Even now, before a crisis, antibiotics that once easily treated common infections are no longer working, and pharmaceutical companies are not interested in developing newer generations of antibiotics because they make more profit by investing research and development funds in maintenance drugs instead. Antibiotics are typically taken for a mere 10 to 14 days. In contrast, maintenance drugs like blood pressure medication and cholesterol-lowering drugs tend to be taken for the rest of the patient's life. This provides a far greater return on their invested research and development dollars.

Most important, I wanted to share my love of herbalism and natural medicine. My hope is that this love and appreciation for plant-based medicines will translate easily through this book and inspire you to learn more. Get outside, go on a "weed walk," identify the vegetation in your area, plant some herbs, and begin to take a new, more active role in creating your own traditional medicine:

> *Traditional medicine refers to health practices, approaches, knowledge and beliefs incorporating plant, animal and mineral based medicines, spiritual therapies, manual techniques and exercises, applied singularly or in combination to treat, diagnose and prevent illnesses or maintain well-being.[1]*

China has maintained its more than 5,000-year-old traditional healing practices alongside a modern biomedical system. The two are not in competition. Instead, the Chinese use modern science to explore how Traditional Chinese Medicine (TCM) works from a biomedical perspective. The Chinese have done much to study and document the antiviral properties of TCM herbs. This information may prove lifesaving

---

1 "Traditional Medicine Fact Sheet," World Health Organization (May 2003), http://www
.who.int/mediacentre/factsheets/2003/fs134/en.

given the emerging viruses for which biomedicine currently has no treatment. India has also retained its traditional medicine, known as Ayurveda, alongside modern biomedical practices. In fact, traditional medicine has been practiced all over the world.

In the West, traditional medicine is often referred to as alternative medicine or sometimes complementary medicine. Alternative medicine implies "instead of" orthodox medicine. Complementary medicine conveys a sense of "in support of" or "in conjunction with" orthodox medicine. Within alternative and complementary medicine are modalities like reflexology, massage therapy, chiropractic care, and herbalism. Germany has led the way in both research and an evidence-based health care system that incorporates natural, herbal, and other alternative or complementary therapies with pharmaceutical options.

Although it might seem that we in the West have no traditional form of medicine comparable to TCM or Ayurveda, herbalist Matthew Wood has pieced together what he terms "traditional Western herbalism" from nearly forgotten folk traditions and drawn correlations between the worldviews of various Western cultures regarding health and medicine. His book on the subject, *The Practice of Traditional Western Herbalism: Basic Doctrine, Energetics, and Classification*, is an interesting and worthy read.

WHY USE NATURAL MEDICINE?

If you're a prepper, you understand the value in planning ahead and having backups for vulnerable systems. You grasp the importance of growing a garden, storing food, and saving seeds for the following year. You have multiple ways of heating and powering your home if utilities fail. You are ready for almost anything—a layoff, severe weather, economic collapse, and maybe even an electromagnetic pulse (EMP).

One area that does not always get the attention it deserves, however, is the medical side of preparedness. What if you were to get sick or injured when professional medical help is not an option? If our medical system were overwhelmed or cut off from resupply, could you care for your own and your loved ones' health needs?

Frequently, preppers approach medical preparedness by assembling a quality first aid kit, then go on to add some bulk non-prescription medicines, such as pain relievers, cough syrups, and antibiotic ointments. Many take it to the next level by adding fish antibiotics. While these items are all beneficial, and I have them on hand myself, there are a few vulnerabilities in relying solely on orthodox biomedical supplies:

+ Supplies will eventually be used up or exceed their shelf life with no way to resupply.

+ Selection is limited to non-prescription drugs, with no plan for chronic illness or severe pain.

+ Antibiotics, fish or otherwise, are losing ground against drug-resistant bacteria.

As part of a well-rounded survival plan, preppers need a renewable source of effective medicines that they can produce and reproduce themselves. Preppers also require a way to assess illness and injury in situations where labs and diagnostics are unavailable.

One way to accomplish this is to incorporate natural medicine into an emergency preparedness plan.

While there are many reasons to choose natural medicine, preppers have unique concerns that make natural medicine of particular value. Here are my top five reasons why preppers need to learn about natural medicine:

1   Natural medicine works.

2   Natural medicine belongs to everyone.

3   Natural medicine is easy to learn.

4   Natural medicine is sustainable over the long term.

5   Natural medicine provides valuable barter items.

NATURAL MEDICINE WORKS

The most important reason to use natural medicine, quite simply, is that it works. It is used the world over because it works and has been working for thousands of years. There are mountains of studies available for perusal at www.PubMed.gov, many of which are free, detailing the effectiveness of herbs and alternative therapies.

NATURAL MEDICINE BELONGS TO EVERYONE

Natural medicine is accessible to anyone. There is no licensing board, and certification courses are voluntary. You can be self-taught or take a herbalism course. You do not require anyone's permission to use or to learn natural medicine.

NATURAL MEDICINE IS EASY TO LEARN

Natural medicine–making methods are elegantly simple, especially when compared with the requirements for manufacturing pharmaceuticals. I don't know any preppers who would be able to whip up a batch of Tamiflu in their kitchens, but I know many who make flu-fighting elderberry syrup in their kitchens. To be clear, there is a lot to learn in order to practice natural medicine safely and effectively. The learning never stops, and there are no quick fixes. People study for many years, pouring long hours into their work. For the beginning herbalist, however, learning the foundational techniques is an easy and enjoyable process with the promise of lifelong benefit.

NATURAL MEDICINE IS SUSTAINABLE OVER THE LONG TERM

Natural medicine's most obvious benefit to preppers is the ability to reproduce or wildcraft herbs, foods, fats, waxes, mushrooms, and lichens year after year. Having herbal remedies to address health care concerns after the pharmacy shelves are picked clean is smart survival strategy.

NATURAL MEDICINE PROVIDES VALUABLE BARTER ITEMS

At some point, people will begin to put a social structure and support system into place. They will rebuild out of a desire to improve the quality of their lives. We can only guess at what any new currency might be. Perhaps it will be gold or silver, but medicines and the knowledge of how to use them will always have market value. Skill sets—such as knowing which herbs can help bronchitis, how to make a prenatal nutritional supplement with common herbs, how to perform lymphatic drainage on a swollen, sprained ankle, and expertise in emergency field or "ditch" medicine—will be sought after.

MY VERSION OF NATURAL MEDICINE

While there are many forms of natural medicine, I have based the remedies in this book on the three with which I am most familiar: herbal medicine, massage therapy, and midwifery. I also include first aid intervention in natural medicine. At the very least, first aid skills are not outside of natural medicine. What is outside of natural medicine is anything created in a lab, anything synthetic, or any ingredient that has been through such processing that it cannot be duplicated at home.

A perfect example to illustrate this point is white willow bark versus aspirin. White willow bark has a long, well-documented, traditional use as an analgesic (pain reliever). It contains a chemical constituent known as salicin, which the body converts to salicylic acid. Aspirin's active ingredient, acetylsalicylic acid, is a synthesized version of salicylic acid. Laboratory-produced acetylsalicylic acid is then administered in a quantity far greater than is available from natural salicin.

Alone, the amount of salicylic acid in white willow bark is not sufficient for pain relief. However, salicin is not the only chemical constituent in white willow bark; it is part of a complex and synergistic combination of chemicals including flavonoids and polyphenols, resulting in a substance whose sum is greater than its parts.

The unique composition of the bark provides the analgesic properties. In other words, you can't simply strip out one chemical, like salicin, and expect it to work the same on its own as it did when it was part of a complex synergy. When taken as a whole remedy—for example, in tea or as a tincture—you feel less pain in much the same way as if you had taken aspirin, even though the actual amount of salicin in the bark is significantly less.

But what happens when you take a substance like salicin and synthesize it? Will such a concentrated amount, which is not found in nature and arguably not what our bodies have evolved to process, have any ill effects? Or will it be an analog, an easy swap between pharmaceutical and herbal medicines? How do they compare against each other?

Aspirin may be faster acting, but white willow bark has a reputation for being longer lasting. White willow bark offers a level of pain relief comparable to that of aspirin, and does so without distressing the inner layer of the gastrointestinal tract, called the mucosa.

Every form of medicine has its strengths and weaknesses. For example, biomedicine excels in lifesaving, heroic interventions and advanced, detailed diagnostics. However, our medical system is unprepared for drug-resistant bacteria, viral respiratory illnesses, and post-disaster sustainability.

I far prefer to see a medical system that allows for all options to remain available: natural, pharmaceutical, holistic, biomedical, and so on. However, when those options are limited by crisis or disaster, it will be natural medicine that is still available for those who know how to use it.

CHAPTER 2
STOCKING THE HOME APOTHECARY

Storing natural medicines is the same as storing food. You will need to designate an area of your home for storage of herbs and medicine-making supplies. This area should have the same basic qualities as a food pantry: dry, cool, and out of sunlight. As with food storage, you will want to rotate your stock.

Many of the items are renewable, DIY projects, such as growing your own herbs, extracting your own almond oil, and making your own apple cider vinegar. If something were to happen to your supplies, you could restock yourself.

Other supplies, however, are not duplicable at home. If you want to include these in your home apothecary, you will need to purchase these while times are good, and purchase enough to last until the crisis is over. Good examples are capsules for capsule making. When stored properly, capsules can last a very, very long time. They are also inexpensive, so you could reasonably stock up on many years' worth of capsules, and in all likelihood, outlast any disruption to services, such as manufacturing and shipping.

FORMULA INGREDIENTS

HERBS

Fresh herbs must be preserved in some way immediately after harvest, either by macerating (steeping) in a menstruum (a solvent such as alcohol, vinegar, or honey) or by drying. As a general rule, fresh herb preparations are best, although dried herbs are perfectly acceptable.

Drying herbs is best done by hanging them in a dark, cool location where air can circulate. Pay particular attention to the formation of mold, and discard any moldy herbs. Alternatively, you could use a dehydrator on the lowest possible temperature setting. Dehydrators shorten drying time, but the heat can damage the herbs if you are not careful.

When choosing which herbs to grow, buy, and store, consider what kinds of health conditions you are most likely to face, and start with the herbs most likely to relieve those conditions. As you read through this book, keep notes on the herbs that strike you as the most beneficial for your immediate needs. You can always add on to your medicinal herb garden or storehouse.

Dried herbs have a shelf life of about a year before their potency begins to fade. To preserve their properties, store dried herbs in a dry, cool space, protected from the sunlight. An ideal way to do this is to place the herbs in Mylar bags with an oxygen absorber or in vacuum-sealed pouches, and store the packets in the freezer.

For specific information on 50 of the most useful herbs, see Chapter 4, Materia Medica.

ALCOHOL

Alcohol is used to extract therapeutic properties from natural substances, to disinfect wounds (painful but effective), and to dull pain. Many people want to steer clear of alcohol for medical or spiritual reasons. However, alcohol—specifically, distilled grain alcohol—is the gold standard for making tinctures. It serves three vital functions:

+ Alcohol carries herbal medicine into the bloodstream quickly, which is extremely important in an emergency.

+ Alcohol extracts constituents such as alkaloids, resins, and balsams that water cannot.

+ Alcohol prevents spoilage and gives your precious, natural medicines a much longer shelf life.

Alcohol has a very long shelf life and is an excellent item to store. There are several categories of alcohol with different strengths to consider: grain alcohol, vodka, brandy, and wine.

Grain alcohol allows for optimal extraction of chemical constituents from the herb into the menstruum because you can dilute it to just the right percentage needed for the specific plant. Grain alcohol comes in a strength of 95% (190 proof) and can be purchased in many states under the brand name Everclear. It can also be ordered online from www .OrganicAlcohol.com.

This type of alcohol can be used for tincture making and disinfecting surfaces and solid objects. You could pour grain alcohol on a wound if you had no other way of disinfecting the wound. However, to say it will sting is an understatement.

According to the Centers for Disease Control and Prevention (CDC), alcohol is not recommended for disinfecting surgical instruments. Although it is antimicrobial, it does not kill bacterial spores that surround certain bacteria. It is appropriate for disinfecting countertops, doorknobs, and other surfaces where germs collect. This is normally done by diluting the grain alcohol with water to 60% to 90% strength. However, at 95% it

LEGAL CONSIDERATIONS FOR HOMEMADE ALCOHOL

Please check all current state and local laws before attempting to make alcohol. While federal and most state laws make it illegal to distill alcohol at home, some states are starting to permit distillation with a license, usually for making biodiesel. This can be a gray area legally, so please check all current applicable laws for the most accurate information on whether home distillation is legal. The ability to distill even small amounts of grain alcohol for medicinal and sterilization purposes will be a highly valuable skill in a post-disaster world.

is strong enough to topple tuberculosis, killing the tubercle bacilli in fluid within 15 seconds.[2]

Never substitute 95% isopropyl (ISO) for 95% grain alcohol in anything that will be ingested. ISO is poisonous to consume. If you cannot get 95% alcohol in your area, instead get the strongest proof vodka that you can find, and allow the plant material to wilt a little bit before tincturing to cut down on the water content.

It might seem as if you're getting an awful lot of alcohol when using grain alcohol, but consider a 1-ounce bottle of tincture. This is the equivalent of a 1-ounce shot glass. A 1-ounce bottle contains approximately 600 drops. The individual dose is likely to be between 30 and 60 drops. So the dose is between 5% to 10% of 1 ounce, which is then further diluted in water or juice when taken as medicine. This is about the amount of alcohol in a ripe banana.

Vodka is widely available at 40% (80 proof) and 50% (100 proof). This range is appropriate for almost all dried herb tincture making. Brandy, made by distilling wine to remove some of its water content, is 50% (100 proof) alcohol, and also falls in this range. Tinctures made with brandy are called elixirs. Wine has a much lower alcohol content, but it is used to make mulled wine. Mulling calls for heating the wine and herbs together.

If this level of alcohol is still too much for you for whatever reason, then your options are either vinegar or glycerin. Neither extracts quite as well as alcohol, and food-grade glycerin isn't really something most people are able to produce at home. I recommend using vinegar as an alternative to alcohol.

VINEGAR

The use of medicinal vinegar is both global and ancient. Vinegar is easy to make from leftover wine, but it's just as easily made from apple cores and peels. This remarkable liquid has a number of health claims

---

2   William A. Rutala et al., "Guideline for Disinfection and Sterilization in Healthcare Facilities," Centers for Disease Control and Prevention, November 2008.

and traditional uses, some of which have promising pre-trial studies in support of them.[3]

Vinegar is an alternative to alcohol in tincture making. A tincture made with vinegar instead of alcohol is called an acetum. Herbal vinegars can be used in medicines, added to the laundry rinse, and used for rinsing hair after washing it.

The easiest way to make vinegar is to add leftover wine to a large jug. Allow the wine to sit long enough and you'll have vinegar. However, the vinegar used most often in natural medicine making is apple cider vinegar (ACV).

There are a few ways to make apple cider vinegar. The easiest method for me is to dissolve ¼ cup of honey into 1 quart of water. Then I collect apple peels and cores after baking something that uses up a lot of apples, like apple pie or apple crisp. I add the apple remnants to the container, cover with a cloth, leave in a warm place for 4 to 6 weeks, and wait for the liquid to turn into apple cider vinegar. Caution: If there are any black spots in the end product, you will have to dump out the entire batch.

Vinegar has proven health benefits. It has a mild to moderate antidiabetic effect and has been helpful to in improving insulin sensitivity. Oxymel, a mixture of honey and vinegar, was prescribed for coughs as least as far back as Hippocrates' time. Research has shown apple cider vinegar to be antifungal.[4] It has even been shown to have a protective effect on red blood cells, kidneys, and the liver in mice fed a diet rich in cholesterol.[5]

Vinegar is often used to clean surfaces, but to be effective as a disinfectant, it must contain at least 5% acetic acid. There are test kits available to test the strength of your homemade ACV. Unfortunately, they are rather pricey at $50 to $100 per individual kit. A decent compromise is to test for the pH, which is easily done with inexpensive test strips. A pH of

---

3   Carol S. Johnston and Cindy A. Gaas, "Vinegar: Medicinal Uses and Antiglycemic Effect," *Medscape General Medicine 8*, no. 2 (2006): 61.

4   A. C. Mota et al , "Antifungal Activity of Apple Cider Vinegar on Candida Species Involved in Denture Stomatitis," *Journal of Prosthodontics* (2014), doi: 10.1111/jopr.12207.

5   Mustafa Nazıroğlu et al., "Apple Cider Vinegar Modulates Serum Lipid Profile, Erythrocyte, Kidney, and Liver Membrane Oxidative Stress in Ovariectomized Mice Fed High Cholesterol," *Journal of Membrane Biology* 247, no. 8 (2014): 667–73.

4.5 or less is sufficient. Vinegar with the proper amount of acetic acid has been shown effective in killing mycobacteria, including multidrug-resistant tuberculosis, on surfaces.[6]

GLYCERIN

Glycerin can be a useful menstruum for natural medicines. It has a shelf life of about a year, perhaps longer if conditions are favorable. Glycerin has a sweet taste and a thick texture, and is useful in making syrups and ear drops. It is soothing to the skin and can be added to cream, lotion, and salve recipes.

Although glycerin is a by-product of soap making, and soap making is a common homesteading and self-reliance skill, making food-grade glycerin at home requires both soap making and distillation skills to produce a pure product. This may be more technically advanced than most people want to get, but if you have those skills, making glycerin is something to look into.

RAW HONEY

If you are not allergic to bees, I urge you to seriously consider keeping bees. Between pollinating your garden and producing honey, wax, and propolis (a resin that bees collect from tree buds and use to maintain the hive), honeybees are an important part of creating a renewable source of natural medicines. It's also pretty fascinating to watch their behavior as they leave and return to their hives.

Raw honey is a miraculous substance on multiple levels. It never spoils, it tastes delicious, and it is an important ingredient in natural medicines. Raw honey is excellent for soothing a sore throat and calming a cough. Enzyme-rich, raw honey is credited with preventing allergies and is the base for many herbal syrups.

Honey belongs in every first aid or trauma kit. A near-perfect wound treatment for everything from burns to road rash, honey prevents infection

---

6   Claudia Cortesia et al., "Acetic Acid, the Active Component of Vinegar, Is an Effective Tuberculocidal Disinfectant," *MBio* 5 no. 2 (2014): 13–14.

through its antibacterial properties and unique ability to manufacture small amounts of hydrogen peroxide the moment it comes in contact with moist, wounded tissues. This means there is a slow yet constant low-dose treatment of hydrogen peroxide directly to the injured tissue. At the same time, the moisture-retaining properties of honey prevent skin from drying out while healing.

Honey can also be infused with herbs to make more specific wound care remedies. Herbs such as yarrow, St. John's wort, spilanthes, echinacea, and comfrey make wonderful wound care infused honeys, either on their own or in combination.

Never give honey or any unwashed raw food to an infant one year old or younger. It could result in botulism poisoning.

BEESWAX

This will likely be the most accessible wax in a post-disaster society, especially after rebuilding begins. Beeswax has a near-intoxicating fragrance and warm color. It thickens lotions and creams, and hardens salves. Pound for pound, beeswax is more valuable than honey and no doubt will be a highly prized barter item.

PROPOLIS

This substance that bees collect from tree buds is sometimes called "bee glue." If you get the chance to work a beehive with a beekeeper, you'll quickly learn why. The bees fill every little hole and gap with propolis. As an antimicrobial, it inhibits infections in the hive. If you place a special grate with holes in the hive, very quickly the bees will fill it in completely with propolis. You can freeze the grate, break off the propolis, and make it into a tincture. Propolis tincture can be used on wounds, but it is also beneficial as a preservative and in giving some antimicrobial properties to herbal products. It is best used in combination with other natural preservatives like essential oils.

MUSHROOMS

A mushroom is a fungus. Mycology, the study of fungi, is a fascinating field of which I'm only beginning to scratch the surface. What I have learned so far only makes me want to know more.

Some medicinal mushrooms are also culinary mushrooms, making it very easy to incorporate them into your diet in soup stocks, sauces, stuffed squash, and savory pies. You can dehydrate mushrooms and store them in Mylar bags with oxygen absorbers. Among medicinal mushrooms are shiitake, maitake, and lion's mane. Unfortunately, the white button and portabella mushrooms we are accustomed to are not medicinal.

Reishi, cordyceps, turkey tail, maitaki, and shiitaki mushrooms, on the other hand, are medicinal. Reishi, one of the most heavily researched of medicinal mushrooms, is both bitter and woody. Because of this, reishi is best taken as a liquid extract or in a capsule. Cordyceps has a flavor similar to licorice, while the others mentioned have rich, earthy flavors more commonly associated with mushrooms. One thing almost all medicinal mushrooms share is a reputation for supporting immune function. The next most common, and somewhat related, claim is that medicinal mushrooms have some significant anti-cancer abilities.[7]

OILS AND FATS

You need oils and fats to make infused oils, which can then be used in salves, creams, and lotions. Currently, the most popular herbal recipes call for exotic fats, butters, and oils that must be imported. Your options are to stock up on these items or produce alternatives yourself.

Personally, I've opted for a combination of stockpiling olive and coconut oils, and pressing my own oils from various seeds including sunflower, pumpkin, and grapeseed with a small home-scale press. If you needed to, you could sprout sunflower seeds, crush them, and squeeze the oil out with a potato ricer to get every last drop.

---

7   Richard Sullivan et al., "Medicinal Mushrooms: Their Therapeutic Properties and Current Medical Usage with Special Emphasis on Cancer Treatments," Cancer Research UK, University of Strathclyde, May 2002.

Lard and tallow are excellent substitutes for some of the exotic butters. Both have a good shelf life. Lard can be kept at room temperature for a few months, in the refrigerator a year, and well beyond that in the freezer. Tallow has an even longer shelf life of a year at room temperature. I don't think I would choose to go back to my old formulas calling for exotic butters now that I make so many of my lotions and creams with lard and tallow.

BENTONITE CLAY

Bentonite draws toxins through the skin and out of the gut. Bentonite works by adsorption. Adsorption is similar to absorption, except that instead of being drawn into the clay, atoms, ions, and molecules adhere to the surface of the clay. The more surface space, the more adsorption.

There are two types of bentonite: sodium bentonite and calcium bentonite. Sodium bentonite is better able to draw out toxins, but calcium bentonite does a better job of remineralizing. I might recommend calcium bentonite for someone doing a seasonal "detox."

Bentonite clay is excellent for poison ivy, poison oak, and fungal infections. In order to use it, you must add water and hydrate the clay into a thin enough paste to apply to the skin, or into a thin enough liquid to drink.

Some brands of bentonite are already prehydrated. I keep these on hand for oral usage, in case of food poisoning. Prehydrated bentonite is a much smoother product than you can get by quickly stirring water into the clay. The clay tends to clump until it's had a chance to sit and really soak. A little bentonite goes a long, long way, and too much bentonite in water tends to clump.

This may sound overly simplistic, but when in doubt about an ailment, slather bentonite on it. One of the most dramatic cases I have ever seen of ringworm uncontrolled even by prescription antifungal cream was treated quickly and cheaply with repeated applications of bentonite clay.

Bentonite also draws out venom, such as from a bee sting. This is something I've had a lot of experience with. Would bentonite draw venom from a snakebite? Maybe, maybe not. That's trickier to answer as there are other substances I might reach for first. See page 151 for information on snakebites.

Because there is no shelf life on clay, bentonite is a good item to stockpile.

KAOLIN CLAY

Also known as China clay, kaolin is the clay most often used in facial masks. It is the key ingredient in QuikClot, which is used to stop bleeding in emergencies. Kaolin clay can be used as a DIY version of QuikClot by pouring right on a wound or by including it as an ingredient in wound powder. As with bentonite clay, kaolin has no shelf life and is a valuable item to stockpile.

ACTIVATED CHARCOAL

Just as bentonite clay has an indefinite shelf life and draws out toxins, so does activated charcoal. Activated charcoal contains tiny pores, creating a greater surface area and more drawing ability. In a pinch, you could use regular charcoal, like the type you barbecue with, but it won't have the "pull" that activated charcoal has. Specifically, activated charcoal is used to draw out venom from bites and stings, as well as infection and foreign matter from wounds. Activated charcoal adsorbs over 4,000 kinds of ingested poisons.

I carry activated charcoal with me in capsules in a bottle. This keeps them dry and ready for use. I break a capsule to apply on a bite or wound. The charcoal cleans away dead or diseased tissue while drawing out the toxin.

Activated charcoal is a good remedy for food poisoning, ingested poison, and intestinal infections because it does not pass through the gut wall.

SALTS

You'll need salts for crafting bath salts and salt scrubs. The salts typically used are Epsom salts, which give the body a dose of magnesium (involved in over 300 functions of the body), and sea salts, which have a high mineral content. Salts are purifying, exfoliating, and renewing.

Bath salts can incorporate herbs, herbal infused oils, and essential oils, which will then be released into the warm bath water. You can customize bath salts to calm the nerves, soothe aches and pains, provide flu relief, and do pretty much anything else you can think of.

Unless you live near the ocean or a salt mine, you should probably stock up on salts. Be sure to avoid table salt in your herbal formulas. Table salt is generally poor quality salt that has been highly refined and stripped of minerals such as magnesium.

ESSENTIAL OILS

Essential oils (EOs) have become quite popular, and it is easy to understand why. They are easy to use and provide a highly concentrated form of plant-based medicine. Essential oils are most often used therapeutically through inhalation or topical application. Inhalation brings the oils directly into the respiratory system, making EOs a good choice for many respiratory infections and ailments. A nebulizing or ionizing diffuser is the best way to inhale the essential oil, but a humidifier could also be used.

EOs are not oils in the sense that olive oil is; they are hydrophobic, volatile chemicals that have been steam-distilled from a plant. It takes a large quantity of plant material in order to get a small amount of oil.

Distillation of essential oils requires special equipment and advanced skills that are outside the scope of this book. However, if you have the land to dedicate to growing the plants and the inclination to learn how to distill them, you will have an extremely potent form of plant-based medicine that will be worth lots of whatever currency is in place in a post-disaster world.

Those who have the resources to grow enough plant material to make this effort worthwhile will be restricted to what grows in their area. Thankfully, several herbs that are high in volatile oils grow in many locales such as thyme, peppermint, sage, and rosemary should be doable. The oils produced by these relatively small planting will give you enough antimicrobial and pain-reducing medicine to keep you well stocked.

Essential oils are wonderful and immensely useful, and I wouldn't want to be parted from mine. But from a preparedness standpoint, there are a few drawbacks that you need to factor in when making your selections for remedies. Here are 10 considerations in stocking your natural medicine supplies with essential oils, especially when compared with stocking tinctures:

1   EOs are not easy to DIY unless you have a lot of land, specialized equipment, and detailed knowledge of steam distillation.

2   EOs are almost always distilled outside of the United States. If a situation arises in which shipping is cut off or severely limited, there won't be a way to resupply your stock of essential oils.

3   Shelf life is determined by the chemical composition and the different chemical constituents, how well the oil is stored, and when the oil was distilled (not the date of purchase).

4   Most of the time, you will not know when the oil was distilled unless you request a report from the seller.

5   Oxidation will eventually cause an essential oil to lose its therapeutic properties. For example, monoterpenes in essential oils have a potential shelf life of 1 to 3 years, phenol-rich oils about 3 years, and monoterpenols in oils about 3 to 5 years. Sesquiterpene-rich oils have the longest potential shelf life, 6 to 8 years in ideal conditions.

6   Tincturing herbs requires significantly less land and plant material than distillation of essential oils does.

7   Tinctures last potentially 10 years or longer. Although some of the plant material in a tincture eventually will migrate out of the menstruum and it isn't possible to get it back in, you can simply shake the bottle to distribute the material evenly before each dose.

8   Tincturing and infusing oils require no specialized equipment— other than perhaps a percolation cone for advanced tincture making.

9 Both tinctures and essential oils require some knowledge of distillation if we face a long-term emergency. Tinctures require higher alcohol percentages than are found in non-distilled alcohols, like beer, wine, and mead, so having the ability to distill spirits would be advantageous. However, distillation of potent essential oils is a more complicated, nuanced process.

10 Tinctures cost less money to make or buy than essential oils.

This isn't to say that tinctures are better than essential oils, or that it's a choice between tinctures and essential oils. You can have both. However, people depending solely on essential oils will eventually run out of them with no way to resupply in a long-term disaster unless they have secured enough land, can grow the plants they want to distill, and can acquire the knowledge and means to distill oils.

The distillation process only preserves certain aromatic chemicals in the herb and then provides them in a concentration not found in nature. This means that part of the synergistic nature of the herb is missing. It's important to pay careful attention to the concentration level, to avoid giving a toxic dose. With few exceptions, essential oils should only be applied topically if diluted. Normally, an essential oil is between 1% and 2% of total volume. For example, if you bottled a blend intended for use on skin, and you had a 1-ounce bottle of a carrier oil, you would add 6 drops of the EO or EO blend for a 1% dilution. For a 2% dilution, you would use 12 drops per ounce.

While essential oils are hydrophobic liquids made up of volatile, aromatic compounds, carrier oils are true oils. They are fats and act as a carrier for essential oils. Always use a carrier oil to dilute essential oils before applying to the skin to reduce the chance of irritating the skin. Lavender essential oil can often be applied "neat" (without a carrier), but most others are risky. Certain oils are considered "hot" oils and should never be applied without a carrier. Oregano essential oil is a good example, as it has caused chemical burns when applied neat.

While not easy to make, essential oils can be extremely powerful when used correctly. Chapter 4, Materia Medica, provides information on specific herbs and plants containing essential oils that may be helpful to you in a disaster. They can be used alone or in other remedies. Aromatic oils have intensely strong properties, making them ideal for disinfecting surfaces and the air. When used in a diffuser and aerosolized, they may be capable of cleaning the air of airborne pathogens, depending on which oil you are using. Inhaling these aromatic oils through a nebulizing diffuser draws them directly into the respiratory system. I would absolutely include certain essential oils for any serious respiratory illness. Beyond their therapeutic value, essential oils can be used as preservatives in natural lotions and creams. The only drawback is that the essential oils most capable of acting as preservatives—such as thyme, cinnamon, and tea tree—have very strong scents, which may be counterproductive.

Recently, I had a case in which the individual in question believed he had walking pneumonia. It hurt to take a breath, and he had a violent yet unproductive cough plus fever and chills. He went to his physician's office, where the doctor ignored his descriptions and did not listen to his lungs with a stethoscope. He was sent home with a diagnosis of flu and told to stay hydrated and ride it out.

While I cannot know if he actually had walking pneumonia, as no actual test was done, this individual did need some help beyond just staying hydrated. So I prepared a blend of the following essential oils, and had him use only 3 drops of the blend in a diffuser as necessary.

Thyme to Breathe Essential Oil Blend

+ 25 drops of thyme essential oil

+ 20 drops of peppermint essential oil

+ 25 drops of rosemary essential oil

+ 30 drops of cedarwood essential oil

After using the blend as needed for 2 days, he began to feel real relief. For use in a humidifier, fill a small cup with water and add about 10 drops of the oil blend. This blend is likely too strong to use with children due to the thyme EO and rosemary EO, both of which should be avoided in children under 13 years old. Instead, use an herbal steam of the herbs peppermint, thyme, and rosemary. I followed this aromatic breathing treatment with my hyssop-based expectorant Respiratory Infection Tea (page 150).

Blending essential oils is an art. Oils are described as having top, middle, and base notes. Top notes tend to fade quickly. Middle notes are next to fade, and base notes last the longest. Sometimes oils are blended based on a number called the blending factor. Oils are further described as woodsy, earthy, spicy, floral, citrus, and so on. Each of these scent groups blends well with certain other groups.

For our purposes, blending oils for medicinal purposes has more to do with the medicinal properties of the oils and not the perfumery qualities. However, using at least one top, middle, and base note in each blend will make your therapeutic blends smell better. I typically use 20% top-note oils, 50% middle-note oils, and 30% base-note oils. Woodsy scents blend with just about any other scent.

The bottom line is that essential oils have their place in your preparedness plans. They are great for short-term disasters, when we may be without shipping for a year or less. For the overwhelming majority of risks, this is more than sufficient. For long-term survival, unless you have a way to duplicate essential oils on your own, it is hard to rely on them for long-term preparedness.

THE HYPE BEHIND ESSENTIAL OILS

There's no mystery here. Essential oils are popular because they are highly concentrated, natural medicines that are simple to use. Essential oils can do amazing things, from getting rid of a migraine in record time to treating a MRSA (Methicillin-resistant Staphylococcus aureus) infection. These are things that modern pharmaceuticals often cannot do easily.

If you have spent any time around the blogosphere, you know that essential oils are everywhere. Articles and advertising are found in abundance in mommy blogs, DIY cosmetics blogs, and survival blogs. Some of the websites do a phenomenal job of explaining how to use essential oils in a safe and intelligent manner. Others, however, make wild claims about the quality, purity, safety, and effectiveness of their favorite brand of oil. You can usually spot these because the bloggers tend to be sales reps for those same companies.

There is a lot of hype and misunderstanding about how to use essential oils safely, as well as how to source quality oils. I'd like to take a moment to clear the air.

Get your essential oil advice from aromatherapists, not sales reps. Aromatherapists are focused on their clients. Sales reps are focused on sales.

If you see "therapeutic grade" on a label, understand that this means absolutely nothing. There is no industry-wide grading system, nor is there any third-party agency that verifies the grades listed on labels.

For those interested in the "essential oils of the bible" trend, the truth is that there were no distilled essential oils mentioned in the bible. Those were infused oils, hydrosols (a hydrosol is the water portion left after steam distillation, like rose water), and extracts, but the technology to produce therapeutic, volatile oils did not exist until the 14th century.

Safe methods of using essential oils include inhalation and topical applications. Ingestion is never without risk. It has a time and place, so I won't say never to do it. But it's rare.

There is no such thing as a "French school of thought" regarding aromatherapy that promotes ingestion, and no "English school of thought" that shies away from it. That's made-up marketing baloney.

Just because an oil has GRAS status (meaning, generally recognized as safe) does not mean that it is safe to consume in quantity. It's one thing to make lemon squares with 3 drops of lemon essential oil (most of the citrus oils have GRAS status) and quite another to drink a glass of water containing 3 drops of lemon essential oil. The drops in the lemon squares are spread out (diluted) through the entire batch. Most people would not eat an entire batch of lemon squares all at once, where they would drink the entire glass of water.

The liver was never intended to process something as concentrated as essential oil. If ingestion is part of your regimen, eventually you will impact your liver.

Whatever you put on the skin sinks into the pores, through each of the layers of tissue, and ultimately into the bloodstream. Take care to avoid contraindications (situations where using an herb or oil would be inadvisable). For example, someone who is already on blood-thinning, or anticoagulant, medication shouldn't use oils that are also blood thinners, such as birch, clove, or basil essential oil.

If a red welt develops from applying an essential oil, stop using it. Redness or, even worse, an open sore is not a sign that your body is detoxing. It is a chemical burn. On my website I have an online course on herbal burn care that covers chemical burns. Be aware that chemical burns are nothing to mess around with.

CONTAINERS

Glassware: Glass is reusable, beautiful, and inert. It will not leach chemicals into your herbal formulas. Unfortunately, glass is also breakable, and I don't know any other way around that other than to stock up on a lot of glassware. This is the glassware I use most often: mason jars for making tinctures; dark amber Boston rounds with glass pipettes and a rubber bulb for dispensing tinctures; and round flint jars for my lotions, creams, and salves.

HDPE: Although glass is the standard, there are times when glass just doesn't make sense. Recently, I've begun using Nalgene bottles for the tinctures in my first aid kit. This is the bag that gets tossed around in the car and on practice bugouts, and I've always worried about my glass bottles breaking. The high-density polyethylene (HDPE) Nalgene bottles are designed to hold up to harsh chemicals without leaching.

Cosmetic Tins: These round, silver tins are what I use for my salves. They can take a few hits, aren't going to break like glass, and can be easily cleaned and reused.

EQUIPMENT

Capsules and Capsule Machine: Making your own capsules of dried herbs, activated charcoal, or perhaps powdered mushrooms creates a convenient way to take remedies that may not taste so good otherwise.

Stock up on capsules, which have a very long shelf life and are inexpensive to purchase. You could fill capsules by hand: Simply take the capsules apart, scoop the powder into the halves, and stick the halves together again. Capsules are great when an herb tastes unpleasant. For example, bladderwrack is a seaweed that smells and tastes awful. It is also a good source of iodine. Capsules make the odor and off-putting flavor a non-issue. Cayenne is another great example. Not everyone enjoys cayenne's heat, but it is a good option to lower blood pressure. Encapsulation allows the cayenne to be swallowed without setting the taste buds on fire.

Your other option is to make a small investment of approximately $15 in a manual capsule machine. This device allows you to fill multiple capsules at a time, and gives you a more consistent result. You will need a separate machine for each size capsule you want to make. For example, size 0 capsules require a size 0 machine, and a size 00 capsule requires a size 00 machine.

Scale: Much of herbal medicine can be done intuitively. Some of it, however, does require taking proper measurements. A small scale is helpful for measuring specific amounts of beeswax, fats, and so on. If you can manage to find a non-electronic scale, great. If not, stock up on batteries.

Mortar and Pestle, Herb/Coffee Grinder: The mortar and pestle is an iconic herbal tool. This simple instrument turns herbs into powders. However, it might take a long time to get a fine powder. A coffee grinder can do a decent job of powdering herbs in a matter of seconds. I have both an electric and non-electric coffee grinder, and the manual one guarantees a finer powder.

Blender: A blender is used for emulsifying (combining one liquid into another liquid in which it is not soluble). This is how lotion is formed. Although you can successfully produce lotion with just a whisk and elbow grease, a blender makes the job easy. If you do have power, either a regular blender or an immersion blender will work.

Wide-Mouth Funnels: For ease of cleanup, I've switched to wide-mouth mason jars. Wide-mouth funnels make filling the jars so much easier. No more spilling herbs everywhere as I pour from mixing bowls into jars.

Strainers: Mesh strainers come in the form of the classic tea ball. Others are in the shape of a basket that sits on the rim of your cup with the inner part submerged in the water. Muslin and cheesecloth can be used to strain and squeeze out every last drop, and a potato ricer does a decent job of squeezing out the last few drops of tincture or infused oil. It's a good idea to get one or more of these strainers for your kit.

Kitchen Miscellany: Have on hand several metal mixing bowls. The types with pour spouts are the most convenient. Also get multiple rubber or silicone spatulas—you cannot have enough of these. You will also need measuring cups and measuring spoons. Some items can do double duty, for example, individual pots that you use for a double boiler. Instead of buying an actual double boiler, just set a smaller pot inside a larger one that contains water.

Labels: I've saved the most important for last. Label your herbal concoctions! Trust me, in a few months, you're going to look at a container and wonder, "What the heck was that?" Always apply a label with the name of what you made, the date you made it, and the date it will be ready.

CHAPTER 3

BASIC SKILLS

One of the most beautiful aspects of herbalism is how easy it is to learn the basic skills of making natural remedies. The following skills for herbal preparations from tisanes to salves are basic enough that almost anyone can learn them in a matter of minutes. The preparation methods described here will allow you to fully utilize herbs and customize treatments based on your needs. Using Chapter 4, Materia Medica, as a guide, you'll be able to craft a wide range of natural medicines, using items from either your local environment or your long-term storage. You will increase your medical preparedness as well as amass many valuable barter items.

TISANES

A tisane is an herbal tea consumed for its medicinal effects. The words "tisane" and "tea" are often used interchangeably, but a tisane is a tea intended to have a therapeutic effect as opposed to one that's simply pleasant to drink.

Plant material can be either dry or fresh. If you are storing dried herbs, be sure to rotate your stock, just as you do stored food. Dried herbs have a shelf life of about a year. Be sure to grow or purchase enough to last that length of time.

There are two methods for making tisanes: infusion and decoction.

INFUSIONS

An infusion is made with the delicate parts of a plant, such as the flowers and leaves. When making an infusion, steep the plant parts in water. This almost always involves heating the water to just short of boiling and steeping the herb for a minimum of 15 minutes. Cover the pot to keep the essential oils from evaporating along with the steam.

A standard infusion calls for 1 teaspoon of herb to 1 cup of water. However, I prefer my tisanes to be a bit stronger than tea intended simply as a beverage. I typically use 1 tablespoon of herb to 1 cup of water. And while a usable tisane can be steeped in just 15 minutes, I often steep mine for anywhere from 30 minutes to overnight.

Mason jars work well to make a lot of tea all at once. I set mine up at night. The following morning, I strain the herbs, return the tisane to a clean mason jar, and reheat the tisane throughout the next day as needed.

Another way to make multiple cups is to use a French press. Put loose plant material in the carafe of the press, and pour in hot water. Place the lid with the plunger on top, preventing evaporation. When the steeping time is up, simply press down on the plunger, which separates and secures the plant material at the bottom, leaving the strained tisane above to be poured.

Convenient mesh tea strainers are available for brewing a single serving. Some are shaped like a ball, others like a basket. I have a basket type that fits in my cup. After putting the plant material in the mesh basket and setting it in my cup, I pour hot water over top and then cover the cup with the lid from my smallest pot to prevent evaporation. When the steeping time has passed, I remove the lid and mesh strainer.

There are times, however, when a cold infusion is preferable. This is the best option for extracting polysaccharides known as mucilage from demulcent herbs, such as marshmallow root. This mucilage is what gives demulcents their sticky, gooey, even slimy texture. Demulcents trigger a mechanism in our bodies to lubricate our mucus membranes.

To make marshmallow root tisane, fill a clean jar 1-quarter to half full with marshmallow root. Pour lukewarm water over the cut root, cap the jar, and let it sit for about 6 hours, a minimum of 4 hours is okay, but leaving it overnight is better. Then strain out the marshmallow root from the thick, somewhat viscous liquid. This liquid can now be used instead of water in making other tisanes. It is soothing to the mucosa and skin tissue throughout the body.

DECOCTIONS

Decoctions are made from the hard parts of a plant, such as bark, stems, seeds, roots, and dehydrated fruits. In contrast to infusions, where avoiding evaporation is important, decoctions depend on evaporation to reduce water content.

To make a decoction, use 1 ounce by weight of plant parts to 2 cups of water. Place the plant material in a pot with cold water, bring to a boil, allow to boil for 10 minutes, and reduce to a simmer. Let the decoction simmer for about 20 minutes (for a total cooking time of 30 minutes). At this point, the liquid should have reduced by half. For a thicker liquid, continue simmering for another 20 minutes or so until the liquid has reduced by half again. This is called a double decoction. I use this double decoction method almost exclusively when making the decoction portion of a syrup recipe.

When you have finished reducing the liquid, strain out the herbs. You now have your tisane decocted from hard plant parts. If you wanted to use both hard and delicate plant parts, you would make a decoction of the hard plant parts first, strain out the herbs, reserve the liquid, and reheat to just below boiling. Then you would add the delicate plant parts to the reheated decoction, cover with a lid to prevent evaporation, and strain after 20 minutes.

BLENDING HERBS FOR TISANES

A tisane can be made from a single herb or a blend of herbs. When blending herbs, I occasionally go with my gut and use a pinch of this and a pinch of that. Most of the time, however, I use the following formula as a guideline:

+ 70% herbs that directly address the primary health concern

+ 15% to 25% herbs that supportively address the primary health concern

+ 5% to 15% herbs that strengthen (tonic) and/or herbs that soothe (demulcent, anti-inflammatory)

Here is an example of how this formulation might work in a tea to help someone with a urinary tract infection, using only ingredients that I can easily wildcraft in my area.

+ 7 parts dried juniper berries

+ 2 parts horsetail

+ 1 part corn silk

The juniper berries are antibiotic and help to kill the bacterial infection. The horsetail is a diuretic that doesn't alter the body's natural balance of electrolytes. So while horsetail does not act on the infection directly, it plays a supportive role by increasing urine flow to help flush out the bacteria. Corn silk, which is the long, silky hair from an ear of corn, lends a potent anti-inflammatory action to the tea, soothing the urinary tract.

This tea could be made even more soothing and effective by using a marshmallow infusion for at least half of the water used to make the tea.

TINCTURES

A tincture is made by macerating (soaking) an herb in alcohol. The chemical constituents in the plants are extracted into the alcohol. Tinctures are uniquely suited to emergency preparedness. They are easy to make, and can last many years if stored in a dark, cool space. They never spoil because of the alcohol. The shelf life of a tincture is indeterminate. However, after many years some of the plant particles can begin to migrate out of the alcohol. If that happens, simply shake the bottle before each use.

Tinctures are fast acting because of how the body absorbs alcohol. A small percentage of the alcohol is immediately absorbed into the bloodstream upon ingestion. When the alcohol is absorbed, so is the plant's medicine. The tincture then proceeds to the stomach, where another 20% of the alcohol is absorbed, before heading to the intestines. This process allows tinctures to start working much faster compared with other preparations such as capsules.

MAKING TINCTURES

There are two methods for making tinctures: percolation and maceration. Percolation is the more advanced skill. It calls for packing a powdered herb into a special piece of equipment, a glass cone. Alcohol drips down through the herb in the cone to produce a fluid extract.

I'll focus on the easier method, maceration. The herbs (the marc) are macerated (steeped) in alcohol (the menstruum), which acts as a solvent to extract the chemical properties from the plant. The marc is macerated in the menstruum for 6 weeks and then strained, and the resulting liquid is the tincture. You can macerate one herb at a time (a "single") or you can macerate a blend of herbs all at once.

There are three variables in tincture making that you must decide on before you start:

+ Will you use the measurements method or the simpler's method?

+ Will you use fresh or dried plant material?

+ What alcohol percentage will you use?

Measurements Method

I'm not sure if there is a formal name for this method, but this is what I call it. If you are using fresh plant material, the ratio is almost always 1:2. This means 1 ounce of plant material by weight to 2 ounces of alcohol by volume. If you are using dried plant material, the ratio is almost always 1:5. This means 1 ounce of plant material by weight to 5 ounces of alcohol by volume.

For example, to make a tincture of dried burdock root, use a scale to weigh 1 ounce of burdock root. Then pour 5 ounces of alcohol into a liquid measuring cup.

Simpler's Method

This is more of an intuitive approach. It's also quick and easy, and I've made lovely tinctures with this method. Grab a canning jar, fill it with plant material, and then pour alcohol to cover the herbs. Run a knife down the sides of the jar to release any air bubbles, just like you would for pressure canning. Add more alcohol and fill to the top of the jar.

No matter which method you use, cap your tincture securely and store it in a dark, cool location. Shake the bottle once daily (or whenever you remember) for 6 weeks. After that, strain out the marc and bottle the liquid. Be sure to label your bottled tincture right away. Please listen to the voice of experience on this: Given enough time, you will forget what you bottled.

The herb you use will determine the resulting volume of tincture to macerate. For instance, 5 ounces of alcohol by volume more than covers the burdock root from the previous example. However, 5 ounces of something fluffy, like mullein leaf, requires much more menstruum to completely cover the marc, resulting in a weaker tincture. The only way around this is to cut the plant material as small as possible, almost to a powder.

Fresh vs. Dried

The next variable to consider is whether to use fresh herbs or dried herbs. My preference is for fresh whenever possible. However, each spring I inventory my dried herbs. Those that are getting close to a year old get tinctured. If I have demulcent herbs that need to be preserved at this time, I prefer to make cold infusions and preserve them by adding alcohol to equal 20% of the total volume.

Alcohol Percentage

The choice to use fresh or dried plant material determines the final variable in your tincture making: alcohol percentage. Plants have certain chemicals that are water soluble and others that are alcohol soluble. Using the correct alcohol percentage is the key to getting as much of the water-soluble and alcohol-soluble ingredients as you can out of the plant and into your tincture.

Your two options are: For fresh plant material, use grain alcohol (95% alcohol, or 190 proof). For dried plant material, use vodka (50% alcohol, or 100 proof) or watered-down grain alcohol.

Fresh plant material still contains water. Alcohol is dehydrating. Using 95% grain alcohol dehydrates the plant and extracts the water along with the water-soluble constituents and the alcohol-soluble parts. Grain alcohol is usually sold under the brand name Everclear. Grain alcohol is also available online (see Suppliers on page 220). If you cannot obtain 95% grain alcohol, just use the strongest-proof alcohol that you can get. But do not use isopropyl alcohol because it is not safe to ingest.

Dried plant material has no water. If you use 95% alcohol, you will be able to extract only the alcohol-soluble constituents, leaving the water-soluble constituents behind. The answer is to use a menstruum with a lower alcohol percentage plus water. You can either use vodka or dilute the strength of grain alcohol with water.

For most dried plants, the optimal alcohol percentage is between 40% and 50%. Certain highly resinous plants require a higher alcohol content to extract. However, the majority of plants fall into this 40% to 50% range. Most vodka falls into this range as well, at either 80 or 100 proof (40% and 50% respectively).

This may sound like a lot of alcohol. In reality, doses of tinctures are measured in drops, normally between 30 and 60 drops in an ounce or two of water. That's approximately the same amount of alcohol found in a ripe banana. If you want to avoid the alcohol, you could add the drops to a steaming cup of tea. Alcohol cooks off at 173°F, whereas water boils at 212°F. Even if you are pulling the water off the heat just before boiling, the water is still hot enough to cook off the alcohol.

To get the exact alcohol percentage, you will need to consult a materia medica, a listing of substances used for remedies and cures. It details their properties, actions, uses, and directions for preparation, including ratios and percentages for tincture making. I have included my own materia medica for 50 of the most useful herbs and natural substances; see Chapter 4.

Let me tell you how I make burdock root tincture using the measurements method. Ordinarily I would measure 1 ounce of fresh plant material by weight and 5 ounces of alcohol by volume. However, the alcohol percentage recommended for burdock is 60%, slightly higher than the average vodka, although 120-proof vodka is sometimes available. The other option is to water down 95% grain alcohol to reach that 60% concentration.

To keep the math simple, I double the amount of burdock and alcohol, and use a pint mason jar whenever I make this tincture. I also treat the 95% as 100%. It's close enough, and I've never had the "tincture police" chase me down for having done so.

I measure 2 ounces of burdock by weight on my scale. In a liquid measuring cup, I measure 6 ounces of grain alcohol and fill to 10 ounces with either filtered or distilled water. Because of the alcohol, I'm not concerned about any impurities growing in my tincture, but I do want to avoid chlorine and fluoride. The 2 ounces of burdock and 10 ounces of 60% alcohol fit into a pint jar with room to spare.

One consideration in making alcohol-based tinctures is that they require alcohol. Home distillation is largely illegal in the United States. Laws change, however, so periodically check your state laws. Thankfully, alcohol can be stored for a long time and can be a vital part of your herbal preps.

ACETA

An acetum is an herbal infused vinegar. Distillation was developed during the Middle Ages. Prior to this, there were no steam-distilled essential oils or alcoholic spirits. Stable oils (true fats, like olive oil and sunflower oil), wine, and vinegar were used as solvents to extract various chemical constituents to make medicines.

Vinegar can be an excellent substitute for alcohol in tincture making, particularly if the plant is rich in alkaloids. Alkaloids are soluble in both vinegar and alcohol, but not in water. The primary difference between the two as menstruums is that vinegar does not have the indeterminate shelf life that alcohol has. The shelf life of an herbal vinegar is approximately a year. Also, vinegar will not extract resinous compounds.

On the plus side, apple cider vinegar, the most popular vinegar for tincturing, is easy to make (see page 12). Apple cider vinegar comes with its own health benefits. And as long as you have apples nearby, you can make apple cider vinegar. If you do not, then raw apple cider vinegar with the vinegar "mother" is available from most grocery stores, and is much less expensive than alcohol. Just like baking bread or making yogurt, you need a starter. For vinegar, it's the mother. The bottles list an expiry date, but I have never found a bottle of apple cider vinegar that's gone bad after that date.

There is no need to dilute or calculate percentages with vinegar. Just use it straight. Make your plant material as small as possible, although completely powdering it makes it a little messy to strain. A muslin bag or several layers of cheesecloth are required to produce a clear vinegar. If you leave your plant material in larger pieces, a mesh strainer will work just fine. The idea is, the more surface area (meaning, the smaller the pieces), the more the liquid you can extract from the marc.

To make an acetum, use either the measurements method or the simpler's method. Remember to shake the jar daily for 6 weeks. A usable acetum can be obtained in 2 weeks, if you are in a pinch for time, or if the vinegar you're making is spicy hot and it has sufficient heat for your liking. Whenever you macerate herbs, such as when you make a tincture, acetum, or glycerite, or when infusing herbs into oil without heat a heat source, the minimum time necessary to get a usable extraction is 2 weeks. At 6 weeks, you have extracted what you can out of the plant material. It won't hurt anything if you keep the herbs in the menstruum for longer than 6 weeks, but it won't be any stronger. If you wanted to make it stronger, you could strain out the spent plant material and pour the liquid extract (tincture, acetum, etc.) you just made over new plant material. Try to remember to shake it daily.

HERBAL WINES

Before distillation was developed during the Middle Ages, there were no distilled spirits with which to make tinctures. Herbal wines, however, were quite common. Although herbal wines are not as capable of extracting the alcohol-soluble constituents from plants, you should explore them as an option for your preps. It is far easier to make wine, especially mead (honey-based wine), than it is to distill spirits.

You can include herbs in the wine-making process itself, or you can mull them (warm and steep them) in the finished wine and then strain them out. This is a type of remedy I personally associate with winter. The wine can be ready in less than an hour with a little bit of heat, but steeping the herbs in wine as you would for a tincture does make for a more effective product.

GLYCERIN AND GLYCERITES

Glycerites are extracts made from glycerin. Glycerin is a sweet-tasting alternative to an alcohol menstruum. Its sweetness makes it a favorite menstruum for children's complaints, and its skin-soothing properties make for lovely herbal ear drops.

Glycerin is a derivative of soap making. If you are interested in having access to this product as part of a long-term disaster preparedness plan, you will need to know how to make it at home. Learning to make soap is a fun and rewarding pastime, and something a lot of preppers already know how to do.

The glycerin that comes directly from soap making, however, is not food grade. It must be further distilled to produce a pure food-grade product. This is an advanced skill, and outside the scope of this book. But if you are learning how to distill for other reasons, such as making your own biodiesel or getting a small amount of precious essential oils, then it may make sense for you to learn how to process food-grade glycerin. It will certainly be a valuable barter item.

For everyone else, glycerin is a finite resource. Once you run out, that's it. Glycerin has a decent shelf life, several years if kept in a cool, dark location. Firm capping is essential because glycerin tends to absorb moisture from the air, and that will change the shelf life.

Glycerin can be used alone as a menstruum, or combined with other menstruums, such as alcohol, vinegar, or water. Because of its sweetness, it can be used to make a strong-tasting remedy more appealing to the taste buds. However, when it comes to digestive bitters, the taste of bitter is necessary to begin the digestive processes. Bitter herbs, such as dandelion root, gentian, and milk thistle, are better prepared with alcohol or vinegar.

You prepare a glycerite the same way as you do a tincture or an acetum. Using either the measurements method or the simpler's method, fill a jar with your chosen herbs, and fill to cover the herbs with glycerin. Run a knife down the sides to remove and air bubbles and make sure that the glycerin is coming in contact with your entire herb. Allow to the herb to infuse into the glycerin for 2-6 weeks, strain out the herb, and reserve the glycerin, now called a glycerite. Glycerites have a shelf life of approximately a year. However, unlike other sweeteners, such as honey, maple syrup, or molasses, glycerin doesn't contribute any nutrients or enzymatic properties to a remedy.

OXYMELS

An oxymel is a blend of sweet and sour made by combining honey and an acetum. It doesn't matter if your blend has more honey than vinegar or more vinegar than honey. The ratio is entirely up to you.

To make an oxymel, take an herbal infused vinegar that has been steeped for a minimum of 2 weeks and strained. Then measure the volume of vinegar recovered from making the acetum and add about half of that volume in honey. If you want it sweeter, add more honey. Add it a little at a time because once you add it, you cannot take it out. Stir the vinegar and honey until they are thoroughly mixed to make the oxymel. As a variation, I often add lemon or lime juice for another layer of flavor and vitamin C.

When I make my version of herbalist Rosemary Gladstar's traditional fire cider, for example, I fill a quart mason jar with onions, garlic, horseradish, cayenne, ginger, turmeric, astragalus, and hibiscus (the last three being my additions), and pour in apple cider vinegar until all the ingredients are covered. I let this macerate for 2 to 4 weeks, and then strain out the plant material. I usually end up with about 2 cups of vinegar. You may get more or less depending on how tightly you pack your jars.

Next, I put in 1 cup of lemon juice, and then finish by filling the jar with 1 cup of honey. You could take this cider in a 1-ounce shot glass or, as I like to do, add 2 ounces to a small glass of apple juice.

SYRUPS

Herbal syrups are sweet medicine made by mixing a decoction or a double decoction (page 29) with either honey, glycerin, molasses, or simple syrup. Simple syrup is made by dissolving white sugar into water. It makes a sweet syrup, but offers no nutritional value or healing properties to the herbal syrup. One thing I have never had an issue with is getting my kids to take their medicine.

Unlike tinctures, aceta, and glycerites, syrups have far shorter shelf lives. The honey in a syrup helps to preserve it somewhat, but after about a month the syrup will start to spoil.

I prefer to make double decoctions for my syrups. It is the water component that encourages spoilage. By making a double decoction, I am reducing the amount of water in my syrup, minimizing the risk of spoilage while thickening the syrup.

You can also make syrups with cold infusions of mucilaginous, demulcent herbs, and use that thick water loaded with polysaccharides as the water portion in a tisane. Then blend the tisane with honey or another sweetener in a 1:1 ratio.

Elderberry syrup, a very old and traditional remedy, has been a staple syrup in my home for many years. It is one my most trusted go-to remedies for the flu, as well as to support the immune system on a daily basis during the cold and flu season.

I use elderberry syrup to make homemade gummy candies, and I also pour it on top of homemade yogurt. Sometimes the lines between food and natural medicine can get a bit blurry, and I think that's as it should be. As Hippocrates, the father of medicine, said, "Let food be thy medicine and medicine be thy food." For my version of elderberry syrup, see Natural Flu Syrup on page 183.

You can preserve syrups by storing them for a year in the freezer or for 2 to 3 weeks in the refrigerator. Preserve syrups with alcohol if you wish to store them on the counter. The ratio must be of 1 part grain alcohol or 2 parts any 100 proof alcohol, such as vodka or brandy, to 4 parts syrup.

If I wanted to preserve my elderberry syrup with alcohol, I would use 4 ounces of my double decoction, 1 ounce of brandy, and 11 ounces of honey. Not only does this very small amount of alcohol provide the added benefit of preserving the syrup, but it also assists in the quick absorption of medicinal herbal constituents.

Other than honey, natural sweeteners that make wonderful medicinal syrups include molasses, maple syrup, birch syrup, and yacon syrup (tastes like caramel). If you have access to some other local syrup, then that's the perfect choice, as it will still be available to you in a post-disaster situation. If you have only white sugar from your long-term storage, you can use it. Although it won't add any nutrients, it will still produce the correct thickness and taste to transform bitter and pungent herbal flavors into syrup with a better flavor.

ELIXIRS

Elixirs are made by macerating herbs in honey and brandy. The combination has a good shelf life, generally tastes better than grain alcohol or vodka extractions, and takes effect faster than a syrup. An elixir can be taken just like a syrup, but elixirs and syrups differ in several ways:

+ The herbs used in elixirs are macerated, not decocted.

+ There is no water component in an elixir.

+ Syrups can be made in under an hour, while elixirs can take 4 to 6 weeks.

+ Alcohol in a syrup is both optional and significantly less than in an elixir.

An elixir is one of my favorite choices for a violent, hacking cough, such as in acute bronchitis. Alcohol creates a warming sensation, temporarily calms a cough, and can also numb a sore throat. In small amounts, alcohol has great value as a medicine. Overdoing it can suppress the immune response. Some people, however, cannot imbibe alcohol. The reason may be religious principle, addiction, or allergy. If you want to avoid alcohol, choose an oxymel instead of an elixir, and an acetum instead of a tincture.

INFUSED HONEY

Honey is powerful natural medicine on its own, without any assistance from humans. However, herbs can add another layer of healing to the honey and create some unique remedies. Honey has antibacterial and humectant properties, and is superb as a sore throat remedy as well as indispensable in herbal wound and burn care.

I strongly encourage everyone not allergic to bees to consider raising their own beehives. There is so much natural medicine in that hive! Bees provide honey, wax, and propolis, all ingredients in natural medicine. At the very least, I urge you to contact your county beekeeping association (every county has one), and find out if the members are selling honey and wax. If so, get to know these people. You will be depending on them and their bee products if shipping is interrupted, and so will everyone else making natural and herbal remedies.

When I make an infused honey, I used the simpler's method. I pack my jar as tightly as I can with plant material and then pour honey over it. I find a nice warm place to let the jar sit for 4 to 6 weeks. Then I strain out the herbs. This can be tricky since the honey is so viscous. Letting the honey sit somewhere warm keeps it on the thin side and easier to pour— mine sits in the cabinet over the stove. I use a large mesh strainer that fits on top of a large bowl, and I pour the honey into the strainer.

Most of the honey will pass through the strainer, but I wait an hour to allow more honey to drop off the strained plant material. Rubber or silicone spatulas make it fairly easy to scrape every last drop of the honey out of the bowl and into a wide-mouth mason jar for storage. Be sure to use a wide-mouth jar because it's much easier to clean than a jar with a narrow mouth. Getting the honey into the jar is even easier with the type of wide-mouth funnel commonly used as a canning accessory.

While honey never spoils, it eventually crystallizes. The remedy for crystallization is to warm up the honey. If I find that a bottle of honey in my cabinet has crystallized, I pop it into a ziplock bag, fill my slow cooker with water, and place the bagged bottle in the slow cooker set to warm. The last thing you want to do is to cook your raw honey. The warm setting on most slow cookers will keep the temperature low enough to preserve the enzymes in the honey.

If you have glycerin on hand, you may wish to add a small amount to the final product. Glycerin prevents the honey from crystallizing. I wouldn't add glycerin to a bottle of pure honey, but it's a smart addition to herbal infused honey. Why risk cooking away the plant properties or the honey's enzymes if you don't have to?

An infused honey that I make in large batches every year is rose infused honey. Rose has a cooling effect on the body, and it also has a profound impact on a person's mood and sense of inner peace. This is something I give regularly to my young daughter, who has made temper tantrums into an art form. Partly from the rose and partly from the ritual of getting something sweet from mom, rose infused honey is often all I need to soothe her spirit.

For preppers, however, it is important to have something on hand to help soothe the spirit after a trauma. During times of crisis, having something to help cope with The End of the World As We Know It (TEOTWAWKI) situation, whether a devastating storm or an economic collapse, is important. In the moment, adrenaline will be high. Afterward, people will likely have some sadness to face. Rose infused honey won't make the trouble go away, but you may be surprised at how effective it can be in helping people cope.

Another use of rose infused honey is as a personal care product. After a collapse, it won't be possible to head to the local drugstore or shopping mall and pick up soaps, astringents, moisturizers, and so on. I have been transitioning my family from all store-bought personal care products to home-crafted ones. This is partly because of the questionable chemicals in the store-bought items, but also because I want to be able to continue our quality of life even if a disaster hits. Protecting our quality of life is a huge factor in why I prep.

You can apply rose infused honey to the face as a facial or as a spot treatment for acne. Just apply with your fingertips, and allow it to sit for 15 minutes. The heat from your body will begin to thin the honey. Wipe off completely with a warm, wet facecloth. This pulls away bacteria without drying the skin. It may be the best facial ever developed for any skin type.

Honey can be infused with sage or horehound for sore throats. A garlic and lemon honey is a wonderful tonic for the immune system, as well as a tasty glaze on chicken. Be sure to check out Wound, Burn, or "SHTF" Honey recipe (page 159) using honey infused with St. John's wort.

ELECTUARIES

Another remedy made from honey is an electuary, a blend of honey and a powdered herb. The consistency can vary from being nearly liquid to being almost dry enough to shape into pastilles.

An electuary may be one of the easiest remedies to make. Choose your herbs for the medicinal purpose you have in mind. Powder the herbs, and then spoon a little bit of honey at a time into the herbal powder. Use a clean spoon each time you take some honey from the jar. Stir well before adding more honey. You can always add more honey or powder to get the consistency you want.

It is impossible to give exact ratios for an electuary, as it will really depend on your personal preference. Mine is for the electuary to have a spreadable consistency as opposed to being a drier paste. I also have a tendency to include powdered marshmallow root in almost every electuary.

POWDERS

You can make herbal powders with a traditional mortar and pestle, plus a lot of patience and elbow grease—or you can opt for the assistance of a coffee grinder. I have multiple mortar and pestles, as well as electric and non-electric coffee grinders and flourmills.

It is not easy to make a fine powder. No matter if you use a mortar and pestle or a coffee grinder, you will end up with some fine powder and a lot of coarse, granulated powder. You can use a fine mesh sieve to separate the two, and return the larger bits to either your mortar and pestle or coffee grinder. In many cases, the only way to get a truly fine powder is to use a flourmill capable of producing fine powders, like cake flour.

Powders begin to break down shortly after powdering. Only powder an herb right before you are going to use it.

Powders are great for encapsulation and any powder that would be shaken or sprinkled onto the hair or body, such as a wound powder. Powders can be used to make tinctures, but straining them is a mess. Encapsulation is perfect for an herb with a less-than-pleasant taste. If you are taking the highly bitter herb andrographis for its antiviral properties, there is no need for you to put up with its bitter taste. If you are taking cayenne for its circulatory properties, you do not need to taste the heat. Encapsulation makes sense in these instances.

If you must store powdered herbs, encapsulate them as quickly as possible, and store the filled capsules in a dark, cool place. The refrigerator is ideal.

Powders can be used for many remedies and applications. Uses include pastilles, tincture making (especially with the more advanced percolation method), electuaries, capsules, poultices, wound powders, tooth powders, and dry shampoo.

PASTILLES

Pastilles are lozenges that are quick and easy to make with powdered herbs and some kind of liquid. Mix the two together, just as you would for an electuary, but let the pastilles dry and age for a couple of weeks. The ratio of powder to liquid will vary depending on the recipe.

Using a powdered mucilaginous herb in the powder portion helps you to form the pastille. Slippery elm is my favorite, as it is naturally sweet, although you could use marshmallow root. If you are purchasing slippery elm, be sure to look for a reputable source; slippery elm is an endangered plant due to overharvesting of the wild population.

In addition to your choice of mucilaginous herbal powder, add one or more herbal powders depending on what you want the pastille to do. Kava kava pastilles are incredible, non-habit-forming mood enhancers. Stress has a negative impact on the immune response, blood pressure, and sleep patterns, and it can do awful things to the endocrine system. Kava kava pastilles are ideal if you are under a great deal of stress and cannot unwind at the end of the day.

For the liquid portion, you have several options. A decoction of licorice root is nice in a sore throat pastille. Plain or infused honey makes for a wonderful pastille. You could also try a cold infusion of marshmallow root to add another layer of demulcent action to your pastilles.

POULTICE

A poultice is a topical application of herbs that have been moistened and applied to an injury. The poultice is usually warmed for low back pain and to relax contracted muscles. However, a poultice can also be used cold on a sprain or when inflammation is present.

I credit a poultice of comfrey leaves, arnica flowers, and lavender flower powder with speeding the healing of a badly sprained ankle of mine. I had taken a serious fall shortly before my mother's health began to fail, spraining my ankle, and I needed to be up and on my feet, walking through long hospital corridors, and ultimately standing at the wake and funeral. I couldn't afford to be off my feet.

Making the poultice was simply a matter of warming the comfrey and arnica in some water on the stovetop, and then adding lavender flower powder to make a paste. The infused water was absorbed into the lavender powder. Once the mixture was somewhat clumpy, I allowed it to cool in the refrigerator.

While I still needed to wrap my ankle and rest it whenever possible, this poultice helped my ankle to heal with reduced pain, swelling, and bruising. For the recipe and procedure for applying the poultice, see page 155.

INFUSED OILS

An infused oil is a stable, liquid fat that has been infused with one herb or a combination of herbs. The process is very similar to the other infusions: Herbs are covered in oil and allowed to macerate. The infusion can be cold or warm.

COLD INFUSION

To make a cold infusion, fill a jar with a dried herb and then fill to the top with oil. If you are using leaves or petals, make sure to pack it. You would be surprised to see how much air space ends up between the delicate plant parts. If you are using roots or anything hard, just fill the jar. There's no need to pack hard pant material. If you are using a fresh herb, allow the plant material to wilt slightly. The wilting is the water evaporating. Water in the oil can lead to spoilage. I tend to use dried herbs to avoid this potential problem, but certain infused oils, such as those made with St. John's wort, require fresh plant material.

When all of the herbs are covered in the oil, run a knife or the flat, plastic utensil from your canning accessory kit (they are designed for this purpose) around the inside of the jar to allow any air bubbles to surface. You may find the level of oil has come down. Top off the herbs with additional oil, and cap the jar. Place in a dark, cool location to reduce the chance of the oil turning rancid, and check on it frequently. Shake the jar daily, or whenever you check the oil. It usually takes 2 to 6 weeks to get the desired strength.

WARM INFUSION

Adding low heat to the infusion speeds the process. I almost always choose to make a warm infusion in a slow cooker. If you have a series of sunny days, you could conceivably re-create the process in a solar over, although you would have to pay close attention to avoid cooking the oil instead of warming it.

A warm infusion couldn't be simpler. I place my plant material in the slow cooker, cover with oil, and turn the setting to warm. Use only the warm setting. If your slow cooker doesn't have a warm setting but just a low setting, you're better off using the cold-infusion method or getting a different slow cooker. Both the "low" and "high" settings on a slow cooker will reach the same temperature. It just takes the "low" setting longer to get there. The warm setting is not for cooking but instead for holding food at a warm temperature. This is exactly what you want when making an infused oil.

The minimum time needed to infuse herbs into oil is 2 hours. However, I typically macerate the herbs for 2 weeks. I turn the warm setting on during the day and turn it off overnight. This allows me to keep an eye on the infusion while I'm awake. I am uncomfortable allowing oil to be warmed when I can't pay attention to it.

Since I have stocked up on olive and coconut oils because they store well and resist rancidity, I might choose one of them. Another option is to choose an oil with specific properties I would like to harness. Grapeseed oil, for example, is valued in skin care for its light feel and quick absorption rate.

SALVES

Also known as an ointment or balm, a salve is a topical treatment made from oil and wax. If you simply warm up some olive oil and melt some beeswax into it, you will get something very similar to petroleum jelly.

A salve is a skin protectant. It provides a barrier between the elements and the skin. Lip balms are very hard salves, whereas the olive oil and beeswax "petroleum jelly" is a very soft salve. Adding more wax makes a salve harder.

I typically use ⅔ cup of oil to 2 tablespoons of purchased beeswax pastilles (beadlike bits of wax) or beeswax shavings from wax we harvested and processed from our hives. If you are buying beeswax, you have a choice of either a solid bar or pastilles. Choose the pastilles—they are more convenient to use than shaving a large 5- or 10-pound block. When we process the wax from our beehives, I melt and pour the wax into small, 1-ounce blocks from which it's easy to make shavings.

The oil can be infused with an herb prior to making the salve. In my Anti-Scar Salve (page 128), which is ideal for burns and blisters, I have comfrey, calendula, and Oregon grape root infused into pumpkin seed oil. I also add some lavender essential oil because I have it on hand. However, lavender essential oil is not easy to replicate on your own without a lot of land to dedicate to lavender and a knowledge of and specialized equipment for steam distillation. If I wanted to, I could add lavender to the other herbs I infuse into the pumpkin seed oil.

Melt the wax into the infused oil in a double boiler, then pour quickly into jars or tins. If you add any essential oils, you can let the oil/wax mixture cool a little. But don't wait too long or the mixture will start to harden before it's in the container. Pouring it into the jar while it's still warm leaves a smooth, professional look on the top of the salve. Wait too long and it will be gloppy and look like someone has already used some of the salve.

LOTIONS AND CREAMS

The skin absorbs lotions and creams more easily than it does salves. However, lotions and creams are trickier to make than salves because they contain water. The water component is what makes your skin absorb them more readily. There's just one little obstacle: Oil and water do not like to mix without an emulsifier.

This is the same concept as making mayonnaise. With mayonnaise, the lecithin in egg yolk is the emulsifier. Technically, you could use egg yolk to make lotions and creams as well, but the shelf life would be extremely short.

Right now, while times are good, emulsifiers are easy to come by. One common emulsifier is called emulsifying wax (a.k.a. e-wax), which is often sold as a vegetable-based wax and touted as a natural product. It's actually a highly processed product that requires by-products of the petroleum industry to manufacture. No preppers will be able to make emulsifying wax on their own.

Truly natural emulsifiers are very few. Beeswax is often called an emulsifier, but it is not. It is a hardener and a thickener, and it can sometimes do a halfway decent job of keeping water and oil together. When beeswax and borax are used together in a lotion (wax with the oil phase, and borax with the water phase), they do function as natural emulsifiers. Unfortunately, borax is found only in a few places on the map, and odds are it's not in your backyard. However, if you live near Boron or Searles Lake in California or in the southwestern United States, and you happen to enjoy chemistry, borax may be an option for you.

Gum acacia is another natural emulsifier. Unfortunately, unless you live in East or West Africa, you're probably not going to be growing the tree this comes from. However, as with borax, you would be able to store quite a bit of gum acacia since it doesn't go bad.

Lanolin, also known as wool's fat and wool grease, is my favorite emulsifier. It works best when emulsifying a water-in-oil emulsion. This means that the oil is coating the water. This type of emulsion helps preserve the lotion or cream a little longer since the water is protected by oil. If you have access to sheep and can get the wool after it's been shorn, you can obtain lanolin by boiling the wool. Keep the better looking fleeces for spinning. Instead, look for a fleece that breaks easily or has an uneven crimp that would be a pain to spin.

To harvest the lanolin, give the wool a good once-over and "skirt" it, which means pulling off vegetable or other matter that may be in the wool. Put the wool in a large pot of water on the stove, and bring to a boil. The fats will separate and come to the top. Remove the wool, which may have turned into a mass of felt, and let the water cool. If you put a large rock or other heavy weight that will withstand being boiled on top of the wool, you may avoid the felting. You will be able to skim the lanolin off the top. You do not need much lanolin for emulsifying.

If you don't spin or you don't have access to sheep, lanolin is readily available to purchase now and keeps for a very long time. Some people have had skin irritations from lanolin, but I haven't heard of this happening with lanolin from sheep, which are typically raised far from pesticides.

Making lotions and creams (a cream is just lotion, but with less water) often involves some kind of solid fat along with the liquid oil. Most of the common fats added are cocoa butter, shea butter, mango butter, and other tropical nut butters that will be unavailable after a collapse cuts off shipments.

After much experimenting, I can report that my favorite substitute for these exotic nut butters is lard (fat from a pig). Lard produces a lotion that is creamy, emollient, and surprisingly non-greasy. I was also surprised that the final product does not smell like bacon. There is a smell, but it is mild, easily covered up by aromatic herbs, and no more odoriferous than unprocessed shea butter. I made some peppermint infused lard and turned it into the most luxurious peppermint foot cream I've ever used. All I could smell was the peppermint. I didn't even need to add essential oils. If you do use essential oils, be stinting because essential oils can easily overpower the natural smell of a lotion.

Lard is ideal for a few other reasons. Pigs provide a lot of meat for their hanging weight, and at a low cost compared with cows. The lard can easily be rendered at home. It can be used to cook, season cast-iron pans, and, yes, make lotion—all as a by-product from one meat animal.

The basic process in making lotion or cream is to take an infused oil, a tisane, and an emulsifier, and bring them all to approximately the same temperature. I use a double boiler for this. I do not like heating herbs and oils any more than absolutely necessary. Optional ingredients include a solid fat and a hardener. Carefully blend or whisk together your ingredients, forming an emulsion. You can do it in a blender or by hand.

You have the choice of pouring the oil into the water, or the water into the oil. I have had better luck keeping my lotions together by pouring the oil into the water, in a trickle, either in a blender or using an immersion blender with a whisk attachment. Once the lotion or cream comes together, do not overmix. Overmixing causes the water to separate from the emulsion.

CHAPTER 4
MATERIA MEDICA

"Materia medica" is the Latin term for a reference guide detailing the ingredients of medicine and their therapeutic properties. The term is used most often with natural medicine-making ingredients such as herbs, trees, minerals, fungi, and bee products. The guide provides information on a substance's properties, preparation, and precautions.

The following materia medica will provide you with specific information necessary for making potent natural remedies. The information I have provided includes the herb's common name and scientific name, the plant parts used, the herb's actions, ratios and percentages for tincture making, contraindications, and some brief notes about the best uses.

For simplicity's sake, in the directions for tincturing fresh and dried plant material, I use the term "fresh tincture" to mean a tincture made with fresh plant material and "dried tincture" to mean a tincture made with dried plant material.

For the overwhelming majority of herbs, the tincturing ratios and alcohol percentages are very similar. A ratio of 1:2 (1 ounce of plant material by weight to 2 ounces of menstruum by volume) is standard when working with fresh plant material. For dried material, a ratio of 1:5 (1 ounce of plant material by weight to 5 ounces of menstruum by volume) is standard. For alcohol percentages, this will depend on whether you are using fresh or dried herbs, as well as the particular herb and its chemical composition. This chapter contains specific ratio and alcohol percentage information on 50 herbs. However, as a guideline, use grain alcohol, or the highest percent alcohol you can find, with fresh herbs. Use alcohol such as vodka or brandy in the 40% to 60% range for most dried herbs.

However, these ratios and percentages are guidelines, and it's best to look up each herb individually, get some first-hand experience making them, and get a feel for how you like them. Or you can use the simpler's method (page 32) and bypass the ratio and alcohol percentage issue altogether.

Like ratios, dosages given are standard recommendations, but not hard-and-fast rules. As your experience with natural medicine expands, you may find a lower dose more effective if taken for a longer period. You may also find that some people need more or less of a medicine. Herbs that are specifically "low dose" will be noted as such; they cannot be increased safely.

Tinctures are generally taken diluted in an ounce or two of water. Certain tinctures, however, may have a strong and unpleasant taste. It is normally acceptable to use juice instead of water to mask the taste. This is not the case with bitters. If you are taking an herb as a digestive bitter, you must actually taste the bitterness to set off the chain reaction that begins in the mouth. I find it easier to take digestive bitters with an ounce or two of something spicy and pungent like Traditional Fire Cider (page 167). It will still let you taste the bitters, but it will be much easier to tolerate.

I strongly encourage you to research each herb further, as there are many additional uses for each. For more information on ratios and percentages, see the Tinctures section in Chapter 3, Basic Skills.

For those who wish to avoid alcohol, consider making either an acetum or a glycerite. You may have to increase the dosage, and there are some constituents that simply require alcohol as a solvent for extraction. However, for most applications, using either vinegar or glycerin will provide an alternative to alcohol for fluid extractions of most herbs. When using a bitter herb, I recommend vinegar instead of glycerin to make the remedy effective as a digestive bitter. Raw apple cider vinegar with the "mother," which is protective of the liver, is my top choice for vinegar in making an acetum. Your ACV must be raw and have the mother for it to be hepatoprotective.

For definitions of all the actions listed for the herbs in the materia medica, see Glossary: Actions of Herbs on page 211.

WHERE DID THIS INFORMATION COME FROM?

We all stand on the shoulders of those who came before us. Over the years I have amassed copious notes from courses, weekend workshops, professional publications, conversations with other herbalists, and books—oh, the many, many, many books! I dream someday of having a dedicated library in my home containing leather-bound books with gold edging—ah... someday.

Also, much personal experimentation (a.k.a. trial and error) and observation have gone into testing the recommendations from these books, articles, and classes. In today's electronic world, there are several quality sources of Internet-based information from respected teachers that have been immensely helpful on my journey into natural medicine. I have changed and adapted my formulas and practices over the years as I acquired newer, better information. I expect that to continue because herbalism and natural medicine are not static. I always give feedback from clients the most serious consideration.

Out of all of this, I have come up with my own materia medica, a rather unwieldy set of binders bursting at the seams with pages in plastic sheet protectors and containing documentation on several hundred herbs and their uses. That level of detail is beyond the scope of this book, which is intended to be a quick reference during difficult times.

On these pages I included the 50 herbs that I think are the most important for preppers to have on hand and that are obtainable throughout most of the United States (assuming supply lines are down and ordering herbs is not possible).

Almost every description of the herbs would ordinarily require multiple citations, but this book would be so unwieldy that it would no longer the quick reference it is intended to be. To balance readability with the need to give proper credit, I've included some references to various sources when the information is quite specific. If I have had a notable personal experience with an herb worth sharing, I have done so. At the end of this book, I included a resources section that lists all the book titles and websites where I did the bulk of my research, and gives additional information on reputable suppliers and herbal education.

❧ AMERICAN SKULLCAP
Scutellaria lateriflora

Parts Used: Aerial parts, fresh or dried.

Actions: Antispasmodic, hypotensive, nervine tonic, sedative.

Preparations: Fresh tincture (1:2 in 95% alcohol); dried tincture (1:5 in 50% alcohol); tisane.

Dose: Depends on the individual. Start with the lowest standard dose of 30 drops of tincture, and adjust from there. Take as needed.

Uses: American skullcap is what most people mean when they say "skullcap." (Read more about Chinese skullcap on page 67.) This herb excels in reducing tension and anxiety. It is wonderful to use when dealing with insomnia, especially sleeplessness caused by pain or nervous tension.

I can attest to skullcap's ability to help break out of the cycle of insomnia caused by anxiety. During a particularly difficult time when my husband was laid off and we had a newborn, I developed insomnia. If you are faced with someone who is trying to cope with insomnia and is full of tension and worry, and perhaps even clenching their teeth while sleeping (and waking up in pain from this), skullcap may be more effective than other sedative herbs such as valerian.

Skullcap can be used in a relaxing tisane about 20 minutes before bedtime, but do blend it with other herbs. The taste of skullcap isn't the worst, but it certainly isn't the best either. My favorite option is to make a calming nervine tea (see Stress, Anxiety, and Traumatic Events on page 157). Add 30 to 60 drops of skullcap tincture to the tea as it steeps. Take as needed to reduce anxiety.

This herb can also assist in breaking habits and addictions, specifically those triggered by stress. Instead of reaching for a cigarette, glass of wine, or junk food, try a cup of skullcap tea, either as a blend, perhaps with peppermint and milky oat tops, or in a tincture added to tea, until the urge dissipates. The skullcap may help ease tension enough to avoid the habit or addictive substance.

During a disaster, I suspect many people may turn to substance abuse as a form of escape. Calming nervines such as skullcap will be important in helping people cope and overcome the emotional toll.

As a nervine tonic and antispasmodic, skullcap helps with spasms, twitching, tremors, and petit mal seizures. This is a remedy I often recommend for pinched nerves with muscle spasms.

Contraindications: May cause drowsiness. Can intensify other sedatives. Taking too much can result in a loss of concentration as well as dizziness.

❧ ARNICA
Arnica montana, A. chamissonis, A. cordifolia

Parts Used: Aerial parts, especially flowers. Leaves are less potent.

Actions: Analgesic, antibacterial, antifungal, anti-inflammatory, anti-ecchymotic, vulnerary.

Preparations: Fresh tincture (1:2 in 95% alcohol); dried tincture (1:5 in 50% alcohol); infused oil.

Dose: Do not ingest. Use topically by applying oil over the affected area or in skin preparations.

Uses: Arnica is indicated for traumatic injury that does not break the skin, such as bruises, sprains, or pulled muscles, tendons, or ligaments. It is also effective on arthritic and inflamed joints. Topical use only is recommended.

Arnica is often used in topical preparations including liniments, lotions, and salves. The tincture may be applied directly to bacterial and fungal infections. Arnica is most commonly used for achy joints, especially arthritis pain. While the roots of mountain arnica (A. montana) are also beneficial, keep in mind that this species is endangered. If you have the option of growing meadow arnica (Arnica chamissonis) or heartleaf arnica (A. cordifolia), please do so.

Contraindications: Do not use during pregnancy. Do not use on broken skin.

❊ ASTRAGALUS
Astragalus membranaceus, syn. A. propinquus

Parts Used: Root.

Actions: Adaptogenic, anti-cancer, antidiabetic, anti-inflammatory, antioxidant, antiviral, cardiotonic, diuretic, hepatoprotective, hypotensive, immunomodulator, immunostimulant, nephroprotective, tonic.

Preparations: Dried tincture (1:5 in 60% alcohol); decoction.

Dose: 30 to 60 drops of tincture, 3 to 5 times daily; 1 cup of decoction, 2 to 3 times daily.

Uses: Astragalus is most commonly used in combination with other herbs to improve immune response. Protective of the heart, liver, and kidneys, astragalus is known as a longevity tonic in traditional Chinese medicine (TCM). It is used to support immune function in cancer patients going through chemotherapy.

Astragalus is an easy herb to add to recipes because of its mild taste. It is almost always used in combination with other herbs as opposed to being taken alone. I sometimes add astragalus to my version of fire cider.

I also add it to chicken stock. I make bone broth in my slow cooker on almost a daily basis to get all that healthy gelatin to my gut. While the chicken carcass and vegetable scraps are simmering away in the pot, I add astragalus along with thyme, sage, and black pepper.

Contraindications: No known toxicity. No known risks during pregnancy. No known risks during breastfeeding. No known risks for children. TCM advises against using astragalus with high fever and inflammatory infections. It's not for use during acute infection. Anyone with an autoimmune disorder may wish to avoid astragalus.

❧ BERBERINE

Berberine is an alkaloid found in a number of herbs, not an herb itself. Plants that contain berberine include (but are not limited to) goldenseal, Oregon grape root, barberry, coptis, chaparral, algerita, and Amur cork tree.

Parts Used: Root. Amur cork tree (phellodendron amurense) has berberine in abundance in the inner bark; it can be easily harvested from the branches.

Actions: Antibiotic, anti-cancer, antidiabetic, antifungal, anti-inflammatory, antisteatosis, cholagogue, choleretic, depurative, hypolipidemic, mucous membrane trophorestorative, vulnerary.

Preparations: Fresh tincture (1:2 in 60% alcohol); dried tincture (1:5 in 50% alcohol); decoction.

Dose: 30 to 60 drops of tincture; 3 times daily, preferably 30 minutes before a meal for digestive/metabolic uses; 6 times daily for antibiotic uses; 3 to 4 times daily for metabolic uses.

Uses: Berberine has metabolic as well as antibiotic applications, giving this one substance a wide range of uses. Each berberine-containing plant has unique properties, and some are better than others for specific applications. However, the various plants can be used in a similar fashion.

In his book *Herbal Antibiotics*, Stephen Harrod Buhner devotes a section to berberine-containing herbs, and lists which have the most berberine. Coptis tend to have the most, followed by Amur cork tree. Goldenseal has the least.

If you use goldenseal to fight respiratory infections, I suggest that you look to other herbs. Goldenseal has a very drying effect on the body and the mucosa. One of my first "trial and error" uses of medicinal herbs was with the misguided combination of echinacea and goldenseal marketed for colds. It was an awful-tasting liquid that essentially was a waste of both herbs. The goldenseal dried me up to the point that I could barely get any mucus out, and there wasn't enough echinacea to be of any benefit.

While goldenseal is a wonderful herb, I don't use it in either my emergency preps or in my herbal practice. It has been overharvested and is now endangered. Technically, if you are ordering goldenseal that is certified organic, then it must come from a cultivated source, not a wildcrafted one. Certainly, if you grow your own goldenseal, you can manage your resource as you see fit. But if we preppers were ever dependent on wildcrafted goldenseal that we had to forage, we would be hard-pressed to find it. It's probably wiser to let that plant recover its wild population and use something else.

Berberine's metabolic applications include maintaining healthy blood sugar, reducing the inflammation of fatty liver disease, improving HDL and LDL cholesterol, lowering overall cholesterol, and lowering triglycerides. Berberine strengthens the gut wall and helps fight obesity.

Studies have shown that berberine, unlike other antibiotics, does not harm beneficial gut flora and keeps candida in check. These metabolic effects are covered in great detail in Kerry Bone's text *Principals and Practice of Phytotherapy*. Many of the studies cited in her book were conducted for 3 months, with no adverse reactions noted.

There is a myth that berberine can be used for only 7 to 10 days at a time. I was taught that berberine is for short-term use only, and I passed along that information in my classes and on my website. However, all evidence points to berberine's safety for at least 3 months of consistent use with no adverse effects. I can only conclude that this myth came about as a misunderstanding based on how pharmaceutical antibiotics can impact gut flora. I no longer consider berberine's use restricted to 10 days.

There is a lot of scientific interest in berberine's multidrug resistance (MDR) pump inhibitor. Just as bacteria have been evolving, thankfully so have plants. While superbugs, such as MRSA, have a kind of a pump that pushes out the antibiotic drug before it can harm the bacteria, berberine shuts down that pump. Without that pump, the antibiotic properties of berberine are free to kill the bacteria.

Berberine does not pass through the gastrointestinal tract efficiently to get into the bloodstream, making it a local antibiotic and not a systemic one. This makes berberine a poor choice for something like sepsis, but a good option for eyewashes and compresses for conjunctivitis, throat sprays for strep throat, douches for bacterial vaginal infections, urinary tract infections, and infectious diarrhea like giardia. Topically, it works on skin infections, including MRSA. Berberine has been shown effective against both streptococcus and staphylococcus infections, but it must come in contact with the tissues to be effective.

Contraindications: No known interactions. Not for use during pregnancy.

❦ BILBERRY
Vaccinium myrtillus

Parts Used: Fruit, leaves.

Actions: Anti-inflammatory, antioxidant, anti-edema, astringent, vasoprotective.

Preparations: Fresh, fermented, or dried fruit (dried at below 100°F to protect the anthocyanins); dried tincture (1:2 in 40% alcohol).

Dose: 30 to 60 drops of tincture, 3 to 6 times daily; in food, as much as desired.

Uses: Bilberry, often confused with blueberry because of its blue color, is known for helping vision and fighting urinary tract infections (UTIs). Bilberry's vasoprotective qualities are especially helpful to the capillaries. More blood and more oxygen in the capillaries means more blood and oxygen get to the eyes, thus promoting eye health and presumably better vision.

Because certain diseases interfere with circulation, bilberry offers some protection from diabetic and hypertensive retinopathies. Bilberry is also a good choice for vascular issues like Reynaud's disease, and venous insufficiency (poor circulation) in the legs.

Bilberry's vasoprotective and astringent properties make it an excellent choice for hemorrhoids. Its astringent nature makes bilberry a decent option for diarrhea relief and dyspepsia. Bilberry is also related to cranberry and contains the same anthocyanins credited with bringing relief from UTIs. The anthocyanins also give bilberry some impressive wound-healing properties. Applied topically, bilberry is according to Kerry Bone, more effective than even the herb gotu kola at cell regeneration in wound healing.

Bilberry is not known to have any contraindications for pregnancy, and is often included in midwifery practices for common prenatal complaints, such as poor circulation, indigestion, hemorrhoids, and UTIs. Bilberry powder is well tolerated by infants with acute dyspepsia (indigestion).

Contraindications: Safe for long-term use. It may dry up lactation, although evidence is thin to support the warning. Possible interaction with anti-platelet drugs when taken in exceptionally large doses.

⅋ BLACK COHOSH
Actaea racemosa, syn. Cimicifuga racemosa

Parts Used: Rhizome, fresh or dried.

Actions: Anti-cancer, antirheumatic, antispasmodic, hormone-modulating.

Preparations: Fresh tincture preferred over dried, 1:2 in 95% alcohol; dried tincture (1:5 in 50% alcohol); decoction; infused oil.

Dose: 30 to 60 drops of tincture, 3 or 4 times daily; decoction, 2 or 3 times daily; topically in infused oil as needed for relief from muscle spasms.

Uses: Black cohosh is known as a PMS and menopausal herb. It relieves the uncomfortable cramping and mood swings that often accompany menstruation, and it can bring on a delayed menstruation.

Black cohosh is used also to reduce hot flashes and bone loss in menopause. Recent research has shown that the herb's estrogen-like effects are not from phytoestrogens, as was previously thought. The effects are brought on by some mechanism we do not yet understand.

Black cohosh has been shown to improve female fertility and encourage ovulation. It also has the ability to lower luteinising hormone (LH), which is associated with a higher risk of miscarriage and is often very high in women with polycystic ovary syndrome (PCOS). Also, whereas black cohosh was once thought to contain phytoestrogens, it actually seems to block some estrogenic effects. Again, good news for women with PCOS.

Considering the prior belief that black cohosh contained some estrogen-mimicking constituent, several studies of its impact on breast cancer cells and health safety for women with breast cancer were conducted. The conclusions were very positive: Not only did black cohosh not mimic estrogen, but it significantly limited the proliferation of breast cancer cells. Black cohosh was not as effective as tamoxifen, but when used together, the combination worked better than either tamoxifen or black cohosh alone. Black cohosh has shown a similar inhibiting effect on prostate cancer cells.

This is an important herb to have on hand for childbirth. Black cohosh can be used to help encourage labor. It is also used to speed along a healthy recovery postpartum.

While black cohosh may have a reputation as a women's herb, it is a wonderful pain reliever for dull aches, rheumatoid arthritis, muscle spasms, and tendinitis. It also has a history of use for tinnitus (ringing in the ears) and rattlesnake bites. No modern testing has been done, however, to verify its use as a rattlesnake remedy.

Contraindications: Not for use during pregnancy or for anyone with liver disease.

❧ BURDOCK
Arctium lappa

Parts Used: Fresh or dried root.

Actions: Antibacterial, anti-cancer, antifungal, bitter tonic, depurative, hepatorestorative.

Preparations: Fresh tincture (1:2 in 95% alcohol); dried tincture (1:5 in 50% alcohol); decoction.

Dose: 30 to 60 drops of tincture, 3 or 4 times daily, 30 minutes before a meal; 2 or 3 cups of decoction daily, 30 minutes before a meal.

Uses: Burdock acts as a depurative. Formerly known as a "blood cleanser," a depurative removes metabolic wastes from the body. In a sense, it helps to keep the body "clean." This cleaning is why certain herbs were thought of as "blood purifiers." Burdock is also a hepatic herb, meaning it has tonic and protective benefits for the liver. None of these roles is surprising, considering that burdock is a digestive bitter.

Burdock can be taken on its own, or included in blends called "digestive bitters" along with other liver-supporting herbs, such as dandelion and yellow dock. Digestive bitters have a cleansing effect on the body because they stimulate the liver. Any time the liver is cared for and functioning at top efficiency, it can bring relief to a wide range of issues, especially skin issues. In this case, burdock can clear the body of skin problems like acne, eczema, psoriasis, and impetigo.

Be sure to drink plenty of fluids with burdock or any other depurative herb. It will help to remove impurities from the body through urine. Otherwise, the impurities may be expelled through the skin, causing skin eruptions instead of clearing them. Besides elimination, the body detoxifies through sweating. However, this can clog pores and allow bacteria to build up.

Sometimes burdock is consumed as a root vegetable in medicinal cooking, and has a long tradition of widespread use from China to Europe in treating cancer, including use by St. Hildegard of Bingen, whose writings are some of the most important documents detailing medieval herbal and medical practices. Burdock has been paired with red clover as part of certain cancer treatments. For more information on burdock and other herbs in cancer care, see Michael Tierra's book, *Treating Cancer: An Integrative Approach*. Additionally, burdock is effective against staphylococcus (staph) infections.

Contraindications: Avoid during pregnancy.

❦ CALENDULA
Calendula officinalis

Parts Used: Flowers.

Actions: Antifungal, anti-inflammatory, diaphoretic, febrifuge, vulnerary.

Preparations: Fresh tincture (1:2 in 95% alcohol); dried tincture (1:5 in 75% alcohol); infused oil; tisane.

Dose: Topically applied in tincture as needed; topically in infused oil or made into salve or lotion as needed; 2 or 3 cups of tisane daily.

Uses: Calendula is used as a tincture or a tisane for throat and oral ailments. It is an important addition to mouthwashes and rinses for mouth sores and sore throats.

In a compress, calendula can help bring down a fever. It also makes a soothing compress for the eyes, especially to relieve conjunctivitis.

However, calendula is most known for its skin-protective properties. It is excellent for all antifungal creams, especially those intended for diaper rash. Calendula is great in any salve for bug bites, scratches, itchiness, scrapes, and burns.

Sometimes, no matter how often you change a baby's diaper, those little tushies still end up with diaper rash. Although my son had no issues with this, my daughter did. No amount of vigilance would completely prevent a diaper rash. The only relief she got was from calendula cream so thick that it was almost a paste. This potent, antifungal cream took a lot of tweaking to get just right. It can easily be adapted for other fungal infections. (For the recipe, see Antifungal Baby Balm on page 185.)

Calendula tincture can be dropped directly on wounds to promote healing.

Contraindications: No known contraindications. You may feel nauseated if you ingest very large amounts of calendula, far beyond what I have recommended here.

❧ CALIFORNIA POPPY
Eschscholzia californica

Parts Used: Flowers.

Actions: Analgesic, antispasmodic, anxiolytic, sedative.

Preparations: Fresh tincture (1:2 in 95% alcohol); tisane of dried flowers.

Dose: 15 to 25 drops, up to 3 times daily; 2 or 3 cups of tisane daily.

Uses: California poppy may not be as potent as its cousin opium poppy. Still, it has some impressive uses. California poppy is effective on its own, and can also be blended with other herbs to great effect for both pain relief and anxiety relief.

If access to resupply were cut off and pharmacy shelves bare, a lot of people would miss their anti-anxiety and antidepressant medication. Now, put these folks who are without their anxiety medication through a crisis. Consider how important an herbal alternative will be for them—and what a great barter item California poppy tincture will be for you.

California poppy is something I include in formulas for serious pain. As a sedative herb, it helps to dull the sensation of pain. It also helps people to sleep when they are kept awake because of pain. This poppy helps relax the smooth muscle tissue, and blends well with corydalis, valerian, kava kava, and St. John's wort.

Contraindications: Not for use during pregnancy or nursing. Not for use in young children. I personally keep this for ages seven and up, and adjust for a child's dose. Do not use it while taking prescription medication for anxiety, depression, or pain relief.

❄ CAYENNE
Capsicum annuum

Parts Used: Whole ripe red peppers, fresh or dried.

Actions: Analgesic, antibacterial, anti-inflammatory, anti-obesity, antioxidant, antispasmodic, rubefacient, styptic, peripheral circulatory stimulant, vasodilator.

Preparations: Fresh tincture (1:2 in 95% alcohol); dried tincture (1:5 in 75% alcohol); infused oil; powdered in capsules.

Dose: Varies by individual tolerance.

Uses: Cayenne is a highly versatile natural medicine. Topically, it can be made into a salve or applied as an infused oil to massage away pain from sore muscles and ease aching joints. Cayenne is loaded with capsaicin, which dulls the sensation of pain. This property makes cayenne an appropriate choice for arthritis, tendinitis, sciatica, low back pain, pain radiating from a pinched nerve, and fibromyalgia. This is one of my favorite ingredients in lotion for my massage clients.

Cayenne is a rubefacient, meaning it increases circulation. Cayenne can be taken either as a food or applied topically to get the blood flowing to the extremities. This can help in cases of poor circulation as well as in poor wound healing, as more blood to the area brings more nutrients and oxygen to the wound.

As a vasodilator, cayenne helps the blood to flow more freely. Taken internally, cayenne can thin the blood. If you need surgery and you tell your physician that you take cayenne as a supplement, you will be advised to stop taking it because it thins the blood.

However, if you are bleeding, you can apply cayenne, either as a tincture or a powdered herb, to the wound. Depending on the seriousness of the wound, cayenne may not be appropriate. Large, open wounds expose delicate tissue. Cayenne can stop bleeding, but it will cause a burning sensation as well. Yarrow is a better choice, but if you have cayenne on hand and nothing else, and the bleeding won't stop, go ahead and use it.

It's not my first choice, but it works. Just remember, internally, cayenne is a blood thinner. Externally, cayenne is a styptic.

Cayenne is hot, and not everyone likes the intensity. You can buy cayenne capsules, but remember that capsules are a finite resource during a disaster and must be stored where they will not be crushed, melt, or get wet. On the plus side, a capsule allows the cayenne to go farther into the gastrointestinal tract before being released. Capsules are an excellent way to take cayenne for infectious diarrhea. One to two size-00 capsules is typical to start with. Adjust the dosage to your body's tolerance and needs.

Keep cayenne away from eyes and mucous membranes. Don't touch your face after handling cayenne. If you do touch your face, odds are the oils in cayenne will migrate to your mouth, nose, and eyes. If this happens, flush with milk immediately. As a precaution, use protective gloves when handling hot peppers.

Cayenne is one of my favorite herbs for cold and flu season. It is a primary ingredient in the traditional immune-boosting remedy fire cider. It is also a highly effective anti-inflammatory decongestant. Not only can the heat of the cayenne cut through intense sinus congestion, but it is also incredibly effective in reducing nasal inflammation. Nasal inflammation is a major factor in feeling congested even when mucus is not actually clogging the nasal passages.

To grow this pepper in the North, start seeds indoors early and provide some heat for the soil. I have repurposed heating pads and clamp-on lighting fixtures intended for pet reptile tanks to help cayenne get an early start in the spring.

Contraindications: Not for anyone hypothermic. If you suspect someone has hypothermia (abnormally low body temperature, 95°F or below), the last thing you want to do is to bring heat away from the body core. After the person has been warmed up and is no longer hypothermic, cayenne salve can be applied to the extremities (hands and feet) to increase blood flow to those regions. Cayenne is contraindicated before surgery, as it is an effective blood thinner. Do not take cayenne if you are already taking a blood thinner.

❦ CHASTE TREE
Vitex agnus-castus

Parts Used: Dried berries.

Actions: Dopamine agonist, galactagogue, prolactin inhibitor.

Preparations: Dried tincture (1:4 in 75% alcohol).

Dose: 30 to 60 drops of tincture, 1 to 3 times daily to regulate the menstrual cycle. Take 3 times daily to bring on delayed menstruation, and then reduce to 1 time daily to establish normal cycle. This may vary in women from just a couple of months and being able to stop taking chaste tree to other women needing to take a single dose on an ongoing basis

Uses: Chaste tree has been used traditionally to normalize women's menstrual cycles. Whether the cycle is too far apart or too short in between, or just completely irregular with no pattern, chaste tree brings hormones into balance for a normal, monthly cycle. This is critical in cases of polycystic ovarian syndrome (PCOS).

In addition to establishing a normal cycle, chaste tree is used to mitigate premenstrual symptoms and increase female fertility. It is also used postpartum as a galactagogue for better milk production.

The way chaste tree works is still not entirely known. For several decades, it was believed that chaste tree caused the pituitary gland to send chemical messengers to the ovaries to correct the hormonal imbalance of too much estrogen and too little progesterone. Another theory was that chaste tree actually contained progesterone, but it does not.

The latest research is both interesting and contradictory. It appears that chaste tree acts in a similar way as dopamine. Dopamine inhibits prolactin. A high prolactin level, which may be due to stress, inhibits the corpus luteum (the follicle that remains after ovulation) from producing enough progesterone. With a lowered prolactin level, the corpus luteum is able to produce adequate progesterone. So, through complex signaling, chaste tree indirectly supports healthy progesterone production.

The contradictory part is that prolactin is a necessary hormone for milk production. At first glance, this should mean that as a prolactin inhibitor, chaste tree should actually dry up a lactating woman's milk supply. However, the opposite has been observed and recorded by herbalists reaching far back into history. It seems that chaste tree—which was so named for its ability to curb sexual desire in medieval monks—or perhaps lactation, or both, still have some undiscovered mechanisms.

Contraindications: No known contraindications, but the traditional wisdom is to avoid chaste tree during pregnancy.

❊ CHINESE SKULLCAP
Scutellaria baicalensis

Parts Used: Root.

Actions: Antibacterial, anti-cancer, anti-diarrhea, antifungal, anti-inflammatory, antiviral, cholagogue, diuretic, expectorant, febrifuge, nervine, neuroprotective, synergistic.

Preparations: Dried tincture (1:5 in 50% alcohol).

Dose: 30 to 60 drops of tincture, every 3 to 4 hours. In acute conditions, double the dose.

Uses: Apart from producing a beautiful garden flower, Chinese skullcap is a potent synergist, intensifying the potency of any herb it is combined with. It also offers some serious antiviral and antibacterial protection.

Chinese skullcap is effective against some of the infections that preppers tend to be the most concerned with, including influenza A and B; hepatitis A, B, and C; Epstein-Barr virus; measles; candida; chlamydia; E. coli; Helicobacter pylori; Klebsiella pneumoniae; Mycobacterium tuberculosis; Vibrio cholerae; meningitis; and various staphylococcus and streptococcus strains.

This herb has a pump inhibitor, just as berberine herbs do. Bacteria and cancer cells that have developed a "pump" to resist medication find that Chinese skullcap has outsmarted their defenses and shut the pump down.

Chinese skullcap is known to reduce inflammation in the brain and protect the central nervous system. It is also a good source of plant-based melatonin. During stressful times, like the emergencies for which we are preparing, expect nerves to be frazzled, immune function impaired, and sleep patterns interrupted. Chinese skullcap can help you readjust and get a good night's sleep (or a good day's sleep if you are responsible for duties at night).

Contraindications: Use caution when taking Chinese skullcap with other herbs or with over-the-counter (OTC) or prescription medications. As an effective synergist, it increases the effect of other therapeutic substances taken with it.

❦ CLEAVERS
Galium aparine

Parts Used: Aerial parts.

Actions: Astringent, depurative, diuretic, hypotensive, lymphatic tonic.

Preparations: Fresh tincture (1:2 in 95% alcohol); dried tincture, preferred over fresh (1:5 in 50% alcohol); preserved juice (3:1 in 95% alcohol); cold infusion from dried herb; topically as an infused oil from dried herb; poultice.

Dose: 30 to 60 drops of dried tincture, 3 or 4 times daily; 2 to 3 cups of cold infusion.

Uses: Cleavers is known as a spring tonic. Use it to support herbal cleansing protocols, ridding the lymphatic system of metabolic waste through urination. Cleavers cools the urinary tract, assists clearing urinary tract infections, breaks up gravel, and may calm kidney inflammation. This herb is useful any time there are swollen glands.

The cleavers plant is almost entirely water (the water content is about 90%). Drying the plant takes a long time, and heat destroys its properties. Try to use fans to air-dry cleavers rather than heat. It will still take 2 to 3 days, and perhaps longer in humid conditions.

It is better to make the tincture from the dried plant than the fresh. The fresh material will result in a lot of water in the tincture. If you have 95% grain alcohol for your tincture making, you should be fine. If not, use the dried plant material with something like 40% vodka. The risk here is that if you use the fresh plant with the lower percentage alcohols, you may not have enough alcohol in the tincture to prevent spoilage.

The preserved juice or freshly crushed plant makes a cooling and soothing poultice for all types of skin problems, including bites, poison ivy, poison oak, burns, and scrapes. You can make a soothing salve from oil infused with cleavers.

Contraindications: Cleavers contains the anticoagulant coumarin, and theoretically it could thin the blood and lower blood pressure. I have not been able to find any reports of complications. Still, theoretically, you could risk a serious bleed if taking along with being on a prescription blood thinner.

❧ CODONOPSIS, A.K.A. DANGSHEN
Codonopsis pilosula, C. tangshen

Parts Used: Roots from plants at least two years old.

Actions: Adaptogenic, analgesic, anti-inflammatory, demulcent, expectorant, hypotensive, immunomodulator, stimulant.

Preparations: Fresh tincture (1:2 in 50% alcohol); dried tincture (1:5 in 25% alcohol); decoction.

Dose: 30 to 60 drops of tincture, 3 or 4 times daily; decoction, 2 or 3 times daily.

Uses: Codonopsis is often used as an inexpensive substitute for Chinese ginseng and even has the nickname "poor man's ginseng." It can help people who are feeling tired or weak, or who are convalescing from an illness or injury recover their energy and vitality. Many books claim that codonopsis promotes weight gain. To an extent this is true. If someone has been weak and wasting away due to illness, then codonopsis can encourage appetite. That's a good thing. It will not encourage a healthy person to start overeating.

As an adaptogen, codonopsis helps to bring the body back into balance. Sometimes codonopsis can act as a stimulant, but not always. For example, while it can be a stimulant and fight fatigue, it may also lower blood pressure. It is sometimes thought of as an immune system stimulant, yet it restrains the immune overresponse in autoimmune disease, specifically lupus. Ultimately, the action on the immune system depends on what will help bring the body back into balance.

Codonopsis is a demulcent and mild expectorant. It is useful in chronic lung complaints, such as chronic bronchitis and asthma. It is not my go-to remedy for an acute asthma attack, but it's useful for preventive care. Codonopsis is also used to address headaches, including migraines, as well as tight, sore muscles.

Do not confuse codonopsis with red sage (Salvia miltiorrhiza), when ordering the herb. While the English and scientific names are easy to spot, the Chinese names differ by only one letter. Codonopsis is *dangshen*, while red sage is *danshen*.

Contraindications: There are no known contraindications. This is my choice for migraine and mild asthma relief for pregnant women and children.

❋ COMFREY
Symphytum officinale

Parts Used: Leaves, roots.

Actions: Analgesic, astringent, demulcent, expectorant, vulnerary.

Preparations: Infused oil from dried leaves; poultice; tisane.

Dose: Topically as needed; 2 to 3 cups of cold infused tisane daily, but limit to 3 weeks. If the injury is severe and requires longer than 3 weeks to heal, take at least a 1 week break from ingesting the tisane, and then resume consumption. Repeat this 3 weeks on, 1 week off pattern until the person has recovered.

Uses: Comfrey is most known for its wound-healing abilities. Its folk names really tell the story: knitbone, boneset (not to be confused with Eupatorium perfoliatum, which is also called boneset), and bruisewort.

Some controversy surrounds pyrrolizidine alkaloid (PA), which occur in comfrey. A study was done using just PA on its own, not as part of a whole plant preparation, and in much greater quantity than a person would take in a normal dose. This type of usage—which is not even possible by home herbalists without some way to extract the PA—was shown to result in liver damage. In fact, there is a long history of safety using comfrey internally.

This may mean that the other constituents in comfrey somehow mitigate the impact of PA. It may also just be a dose-dependent reaction. In either case, there is more PA found in the root than the leaf. If you are looking to avoid PA, then avoid the root and stick to the leaves.

Personally, I rarely make a tincture of comfrey, although I have some on hand. For most purposes, I favor an infusion made from dried leaves for internal use. Comfrey is also wonderful in salves. You will find salve recipes that include comfrey in Chapter 5, Herbal First Aid Kit. Use comfrey salve for bug bites, blisters, scrapes, bruises, and comfrey poultices for sprains, and fractures.

Comfrey poultices are a must-have for lower back pain, and to help bones, tendons, and ligaments heal. Make a cold infusion of comfrey, and without straining the leaves, mix in flour or a powder to form a paste. I use lavender flower powder, but even bread flour will work. Spread the poultice on the injured site, and, if possible, wrap to keep in place. Or you could put the paste in a muslin bag and then apply it to the injury.

The one caution I stress is that comfrey is so efficient at wound healing and cell regeneration that it is not for use in deep wounds. Comfrey will heal the top layers too fast, and healing a wound from the outside in is the last thing you want for a puncture or other deep wound. That could easily leave the wound underneath vulnerable to infection. St. John's wort and honey are much better choices for a deep wound.

Contraindications: Not for use during pregnancy or breastfeeding. Not for long-term use. Not for use on people with liver disease. Use with children should be limited and the dose adjusted. See instructions on calculating children's dosage on page 122.

❦ CRAMP BARK
Viburnum opulus

Parts Used: Bark.

Actions: Astringent, anti-inflammatory, antispasmodic, nervine.

Preparations: Dried tincture (1:5 in 50% alcohol); strong decoction.

Dose: 30 to 90 drops, 3 or 4 times daily; 3 to 4 cups of strong decoction daily.

Uses: Cramp bark is used to relieve muscle cramping and spasms. It is widely used for cramping associated with PMS. If excessive bleeding is a problem during menstruation, cramp bark's astringent nature may help to rein it in. Cramp bark, along with other herbs, is used by midwives for cramping and bleeding during pregnancy, and when miscarriage is a risk.

Cramp bark can be helpful with any kind of spasm, not just spasms associated with the uterus. It can be used to help relieve asthma, violent coughing from bronchitis, or a muscle spasm. Like another viburnum, Black haw *(V. prunifolum),* cramp bark contains two antispasmodic phytochemicals, aesculetin and scopoletin. Cramp bark also has a small amount of salicin, which is related to the synthetic acetylsalicylic acid, or aspirin.

Contraindications: Not for anyone with a history of kidney stones. Not for anyone allergic to aspirin. While there is no evidence to show that salicin would cause the same reaction as acetylsalicylic acid, there is no evidence to show that it wouldn't. Do not give cramp bark to children with a fever. Cramp bark may worsen tinnitus.

❦ DANDELION
Taraxacum officinale

Parts Used: Fresh or dried root, fresh leaves, fresh flowers.

Actions: Antirheumatic, bitter, cholagogue, choleretic, diuretic, tonic.

Preparations: Fresh tincture from root or entire plant (1:2 in 75% alcohol); dried tincture from root (1:5 in 50% alcohol); tisane from fresh flowers; infused oil from fresh flowers; wine from fresh flowers; fresh leaves added to salads and soups.

Dose: 30 to 60 drops of tincture, 3 or 4 times daily; tisane, 2 or 3 times daily; fresh leaves freely as food; dandelion wine in moderation.

Uses: Dandelion is bitter, tonic, and diuretic. It is used as a tonic after winter's long digestive slumber without fresh foods. Dandelion root tincture kick-starts digestion; it revs up the liver's bile production and encourages bile to move deeper into the digestive system. Bile is necessary for the proper absorption of fats and nutrients, as well as the elimination of wastes from the body.

Dandelion is a highly effective diuretic. However, unlike many diuretics, dandelion is high in potassium and replenishes potassium lost in urination.

Look to digestive bitters to help anyone who has been taking large amounts of pharmaceuticals, alcohol, or processed foods; lacks sufficient vegetables in the diet; has an hormonal imbalance, skin condition, urinary tract infection, or fatty liver disease; is overweight; or has insulin resistance. Dandelion is in almost every bitters blend I make. If the liver needs something gentler, I might look to soups with dandelion greens, or a tincture made from the leaves and flowers instead of the more potent roots.

Contraindications: Not for anyone with gallstones, or any inflammation or disease of the gallbladder.

❧ ECHINACEA
Echinacea angustifolia, E. purpurea

Parts Used: Root of *E. angustifolia*; aerial parts of *E. purpurea;* seeds of either species.

Actions: Analgesic, antibiotic, anti-inflammatory, antiviral, immuno-stimulant, vulnerary.

Preparations: Fresh tincture from *E. angustifolia* (1:2 in 95% alcohol); dried tincture from *E. angustifolia* (1:5 in 70% alcohol); *E. purpurea* is best made into juice and preserved (3:1 with 95% alcohol); seeds (1:4 in 75% alcohol); wound powder.

Dose: 30 to 60 drops of root or seed tincture, 3 to 6 times daily for topical infections; in acute illness, 30 drops every 30 minutes; 1 ounce of *E. purpurea* juice, 3 to 6 times daily; topically as wound powder, as needed.

Uses: Echinacea is probably one of the most misunderstood and misused herbs. It is most commonly known as a cold and flu preventive and treatment, which is a fairly poor use of it. Some people say usage must be kept under 7 days and others say 3 weeks, and yet the Eclectic physicians, America's forgotten physicians who used botanical medicines extensively, used echinacea for much longer periods and never mentioned a time limitation. Other people insist that echinacea is an immune "tonic," which it is not. And the worst are those claiming echinacea is a cure-all.

Echinacea is not an immune tonic. That would mean it supports and strengthens the immune system. That's not what echinacea does. Echinacea stimulates immune response. Stimulating a system to work more and work harder is different from building up and supporting a system.

A cautionary note: If you do not rest and focus on proper recuperation, and instead rely on echinacea to force your way through an infection, ultimately your immune system will be too spent and a far more serious case of infection will result.

To be clear, it's not that echinacea won't help a cold or the flu, but rather that it's not what this herb really excels at and there are better herbs for that purpose. If you are going to use echinacea for a cold, then you must take it right at the onset of symptoms, and take hefty, frequent doses of it. If that's what you have on hand, use it. However, there are more effective ways to approach a cold or flu that don't involve using echinacea tincture every half hour.

When taking echinacea tincture orally, it's best to take it sublingually. Place the drops under the tongue, and hold them there for approximately 1 minute. This helps to get the herb into the bloodstream as quickly as possible. Adding echinacea to water diminishes its effectiveness.

Echinacea creates a numbing sensation, making it appropriate for sore throat sprays, children's ear oils, and topical application either through tincture, powder, or salve made from echinacea infused oil. During an emergency when no medical help is available, echinacea tincture can be used topically on venomous bites by dropping 30 to 60 drops of tincture directly on the bite. For more on dealing with bites, see "Snake- and Spider-Bite" Care on page 151.

Echinacea is an excellent ingredient in wound powders as it helps to numb the sensation of pain and is also being antibacterial. These same properties make the tincture a good option for dental abscesses and other oral wounds.

Echinacea is systemic if given in very large doses, meaning it can enter the bloodstream. Because echinacea is able to enter the bloodstream, it can be added to other herbal formulas to treat septicemia, or blood poisoning. Septicemia can lead to sepsis, a very dangerous condition in which the entire body responds to an infection somewhere in the body. Sepsis can lead to multi-organ failure.

Echinacea makes for a lousy-tasting tea, but a tisane or decoction made from it can be used as a wound wash.

Echinacea has a history of safe usage among pregnant and nursing women when using the recommended dosage and for short periods of time. There doesn't seem to be any toxicity or reason to expect problems from long-term use. However, at the time of this writing, there are no controlled studies of pregnant or nursing women who have taken echinacea on a long-term basis.

Contraindications: If you are allergic to ragweed, you may have an allergic reaction to echinacea. It isn't a guarantee, as I know several people who are allergic to ragweed and have no ill response from echinacea. Another point of confusion is with autoimmune diseases. Echinacea is an immunostimulant. With as many people as we have today diagnosed with autoimmune diseases and with an herb so commonly consumed as echinacea, you would expect to see ample evidence of harmful reactions to echinacea consumption. In fact, that isn't the case. To anyone with an autoimmune disease who wants to try echinacea, I suggest proceeding with caution and common sense.

❧ ELDER
Sambucus nigra canadensis

Parts Used: Berries, flowers; rarely leaves and roots (see comments on leaves and roots below).

Actions: Antibacterial, antiviral, immunostimulant.

Preparations: Dried tincture from berries (1:4 in 60% alcohol); fresh tincture from flowers (1:2 in 75% alcohol); dried tincture from flowers (1:5 in 50% alcohol); fresh berries in syrup and prepared foods (such as preserves and pie fillings).

Dose: 30 to 60 drop of tincture, 3 to 6 times daily; 1 teaspoon of syrup (minimum) throughout the day.

Uses: While the berries and flowers are effective against a limited range of bacteria, and the roots and leaves have emetic properties, elder is known for its berries because they does one thing exceptionally well: They fight the flu. The combination of both elderberry and elder flower make, in my opinion, a stronger medicine together than separately. There is ample research on the safety and efficacy of elderberry as a remedy for various strains of both influenza A and B.

Unfortunately, elder is not effective on rhinovirus, the virus most often behind the common cold. While elderberry is not a remedy for the common cold, both the berry and flower are immunostimulants. Although this herb does not work directly on a cold, it can be taken to increase immune response.

Elderberry syrup—a delicious, warming syrup with a honey base—is an easy, tasty remedy for respiratory issues I have been making for years (see Natural Flu Syrup on page 183). Kids love it and will ask for more. I give 1 teaspoon every hour for the first day. Then I back down to every 2 to 3 hours the next day, and continue until symptoms stop. It may sound like a lot of syrup, but it's tasty. I add it as a topping to homemade yogurt. (Also, I do not wait until it's obvious whether the respiratory infection is a cold or the flu. See entry on Ginger.)

The tincture can be taken with honey and brandy as an elixir. Instead, I usually opt to add it to a glass of apple juice. If I have apple cider on hand, even better. The flavors go well together and encourage the consumption of fluids, which is important during the flu.

Topically, tinctures made from the root and leaves are antifungal. See Contraindications below for more information on elderberry root and leaves.

Contraindications: There are some misconceptions about elder's safety and toxicity. Elder root and leaves, as well as the uncooked berries to a lesser degree, are emetic. This means, if you take enough of these plant parts, they will induce vomiting. However, this is not quite the same thing as being poisonous. Emetics are used to induce vomiting, which may be useful in case of a poisoning. If you have been poisoned, and have any option at all of getting to a doctor, do so immediately. If that is not an option, emetic herbs may be appropriate. Topically, the roots mashed into a poultice are safe to use on stubborn fungal infections.

❊ ELECAMPANE
Inula helenium

Parts Used: Root.

Actions: Antimicrobial, antitussive, demulcent, diaphoretic, diuretic, expectorant, vermifuge.

Preparations: Fresh tincture (1:2 in 75% alcohol); dried tincture (1:5 in 50% alcohol); cold infusion; decoction; syrup; candied root; powdered root pastilles; infused honey.

Dose: As needed for relief from deep or lingering coughs; 30 to 60 drops of tincture daily to expel parasitic worms.

Uses: Elecampane is a powerful remedy for tough coughs and tightness in the chest. When difficulty in breathing is the problem, I reach for elecampane. In the tincture, the alcohol portion extracts antimicrobial properties, while the water portion extracts the polysaccharides that make elecampane a superior herb for respiratory complaints.

Elecampane is bitter, but not very bitter. It can be sweetened easily enough with honey, which has the benefit of soothing a sore throat. Elecampane can be made into a syrup, infused honey, or powdered and made into pastilles with honey.

As an expectorant, elecampane can be included in remedies for asthma, whooping cough, and shortness of breath. The 17th-century herbalist Nicholas Culpepper wrote that elecampane could be chewed or made into a tea to gargle to reset loose teeth and prevent the teeth from "putrefaction."

Contraindications: Not for use while pregnant or breastfeeding. Tea, syrup, and candied elecampane can be taken by children who are over one year of age.

❦ GARLIC
Allium sativum

Parts Used: Bulb.

Actions: Antibacterial, choleretic, diaphoretic, expectorant, hypotensive, immunotonic, immunostimulant, vasodilator, vulnerary.

Preparations: Raw or lacto-fermented whole cloves according to taste; fresh tincture of raw cloves (1:2 in 95% alcohol), 3 to 4 times daily; decoction 2 to 3 times daily; 1 teaspoon syrup, 3 to 6 times daily; infused oil for use as ear drops, 1 to 2 drops in ear as needed.

Dose: 30 to 60 drops of tincture, 3 to 4 times daily; consume to taste and stomach tolerance in diet; due to garlic's strong, pungent flavor, it is the individual's personal tastes which will dictate how much garlic to include in a remedy such as a decoction or syrup or with food.

Uses: Garlic benefits the immune system, respiratory system, and circulatory system. It is associated with lower cancer risks and can be applied in topical preparations as an antibiotic. In World War II, soldiers used garlic juice as a topical treatment to prevent wounds from becoming infected and worsening into septicemia (bacteria in the blood) or sepsis (when bacteria has infected an organ). Ingested, garlic acts as an immunotonic, strengthening the immune system, and as an immunostimulant to kick-start immune response when an infection begins to take hold.

Garlic works especially well for respiratory infections. Garlic taken as a tincture, decoction, syrup, or in the diet, perhaps in soup or a strong, garlicky tomato sauce, right at the beginning of a cold can often stop the cold in its tracks. This is assuming, however, that the sick person takes the time to properly rest and let the body handle the infection. Garlic induces sweating. Open pores for perspiration is one of the ways the body detoxifies itself. Inducing perspiration is cooling, and the most beneficial way for the body to reduce a fever.

Choleretics are a good choice to help the liver when it may be a bit overworked. Garlic's function as a choleretic means it triggers the body to produce more bile, which helps the liver work more efficiently. For example, if you have taken a lot of prescription drugs, that's a lot of strain on the liver. It is the liver's job to filter out what is helpful and what is toxic to the body. When overworked, the liver may not be filtering as efficiently as it should. The same is true for certain hormonal imbalances where excess hormones are filtered out by the liver. At some point, the liver becomes sluggish and does not do a good job as the body's filter. Choleretics, many of which are strong-tasting, bitter, or pungent herbs, help the body help the liver get the job done.

Last but not least, garlic is widely used to improve heart and circulatory health. Garlic encourages vasodilation, which expands the blood vessels

WHAT IS LACTO-FERMENTATION?

Lacto-fermentation is a process that uses beneficial bacteria to ferment foods, as opposed to using a yeast as is done for breads, beer, and wine. The "lacto" in lacto-fermentation comes from "lactobacillus," a genus of bacteria with several species, like L. acidophilus and L. reuteri. These types of bacteria are found naturally on plant surfaces and help to keep a healthy balance of bacteria in our intestines.

During the fermentation process, a small amount of salt prevents spoilage just long enough to allow the beneficial bacteria to flourish and get the fermentation process going. Whey can be added with or instead of salt, as it provides the needed levels of bacteria right from the beginning. Whey is a by-product of making yogurt, which is also made by lacto-fermentation, just without the salt. During the fermentation process, the nutrients are made more bioavailable, so you get more nutrients from your food. The process also reduces the amount of gluten if present.

Common ferments are cabbage (sauerkraut), kimchi, yogurt, kefir, and sourdough bread. Just about any vegetable can be fermented this way, and can be stored for many months in cool temperatures without refrigeration, such as a root cellar or basement. Fermented dairy does still require refrigeration.

and thereby lowers blood pressure. It is used to prevent hardened arteries. When arteries harden, the body tries to heal over the area with cholesterol. The body uses cholesterol to protect the blood vessel, like a soothing balm over a scab. Unfortunately, this can also cause a blockage if too much cholesterol collects in one spot.

Garlic and other circulatory and heart-healthy herbs are best used in a preventative way to cultivate heart health, as opposed to a response to a cardiovascular emergency. Unfortunately, there are no good answers for a cardiac emergency without access to a hospital. Herbs and natural remedies can offer great preventative care as well as solid aftercare. But, if one were to have a heart attack when no hospital care is available, the best thing to do is to just relax through it. Someone must be designated as the heath care provider, ideally with assistants, and that person must be able to administer CPR. It would be very beneficial to have a portable defibrillator (AED machine) for your family or mutual support group, and have someone trained on how to use it.

The moral of this story is to eat garlic. Eat it raw. Eat if fermented. Eat it cooked. It's good for you any way you take it. Garlic is both a medicinal herb as well as a food. There is no maximum "dosage" other than your own taste buds can handle, and there is potentially some stomach upset if you eat too much.

Finally, there is one more garlic remedy that needs to be discussed— garlic infused oil. This is an old remedy for ear infections. It's simple and effective, and if you can warm garlic in oil, you can soothe a child's earache quickly. The tricky part about making garlic infused oil is that it is very easy to end up with botulism in your oil, especially when macerating garlic in oil for weeks at a time.

With other herbs, I normally let my oils infuse anywhere from 2 hours to 2 weeks in a slow cooker. (A well-vented solar oven would work as a substitute for a slow cooker where there is no electricity.) But, with garlic, I let this warm up gently anywhere from 2 to 6 hours tops, and then strain out the garlic, which I would likely use to make chili that night or some hummus for a snack. Then, I store my garlic infused oil in the freezer for safety. Botulism can grow anywhere between 40° and 120°F. Most refrigerators are set for 40°F, but if power were to go out, a well-packed freezer will retain its colder temperatures longer. Freeze it in ice cube trays, and when solid, transfer to a freezer storage bag. When you need it, just take a cube out and let it melt. I store this in small, glass jars which can be gently warmed by putting the jar in warm water. Use an eye dropper to dispense.

If electricity is out and freezer storage is not possible, then only make garlic oil in micro-batches of just enough for your needs at the moment. Other options for earache oils would be mullein flower, bee balm (Monarda fistulosa), and echinacea glycerite.

Many people have stored garlic cloves in oil on the counter and never had an issue. That still doesn't make is safe. Botulism is a serious medical emergency in the best of times. A little extra precaution to prevent it in the worst of times seems prudent.

Contraindications: When breastfeeding, garlic may cause gastric upset (nausea or heartburn) in the infant. Gastric upset can also occur in adults eating very large amounts of raw garlic.

❦ GINGER
Zingiber officinale

Parts Used: Rhizome (almost always referred to as a root).

Actions: Analgesic, anti-arthritic, antibacterial, anti-diarrhea, anti-emetic, anti-inflammatory, antifungal, antispasmodic, antitussive, antiviral, diaphoretic, hypotensive, immunostimulant, peripheral circulatory stimulant, synergistic vasodilator.

Preparations: Fresh tincture (1:2 in 95% alcohol); preserved juice (3:1 in 95% alcohol); decoction; syrup; infused honey; candied ginger.

Dose: Depends on individual taste, take as needed.

Uses: Ginger is a must-have natural medicine. Even if you live in a cold climate, ginger is worth growing in containers and bringing indoors for the winter. It is a potent synergist, making a blend of herbs more powerful than each herb on its own. Ginger is excellent for viral respiratory infections, pain relief, and gastrointestinal problems.

The very first medicinal herbal remedy I ever tried was a very strong-flavored decoction heavy with ginger. I had the flu, and it was rough going. The ginger caused me to sweat, helped to calm the violent coughing, and chased away the aches and the chill of the flu. I was better in record time, just a matter of days. It was my "aha" moment with herbs and natural medicines.

I have used ginger successfully to reduce inflammation in swollen joints from a host of complaints—everything from arthritic joints to swelling triggered by food allergies.

Ginger has shown effectiveness against the common cold (rhinovirus), whereas elderberry has not—but elderberry fights the flu. The two tastes blend very well together. Rather than wait and see if the infection is a cold or the flu, take a syrup combining elderberry and ginger (and other ingredients, including echinacea) at the first sniffle.

For nausea and the horrible stomach cramping associated with bouts of diarrhea, ginger is an important herbal ally. It acts against E. coli, salmonella, listeria, and Helicobacter pylori bacteria.

Ginger is a well-known remedy for morning sickness in pregnant women. Despite a pervasive myth that ginger will trigger a miscarriage, there is no evidence that ginger does any such thing.

As a peripheral circulatory stimulant, ginger brings blood to the extremities. That means ginger will help in cases of cold weather injuries to the hands or feet. Give the ginger with cayenne (also a peripheral circulatory stimulant), but only after making sure that the core of the body is sufficiently warm.

Contraindications: In high doses, ginger may thin the blood and cause heartburn. Ginger is a synergist, so it may increase the effect of medication taken with it. If pregnant, avoid excessively large amounts of ginger.

❦ GOLDENROD
Solidago canadensis

Parts Used: Flowers, leaves.

Actions: Analgesic, anti-allergenic, anti-inflammatory, astringent, diaphoretic, diuretic, expectorant, renal trophorestorative.

Preparations: Fresh tincture (1:2 in 75% alcohol); dried tincture (1:5 in 50% alcohol); cold infusion; standard infusion tisane; infused oil; acetum; elixir.

Dose: 30 to 60 drops of tincture, elixir, or acetum, 3 or 4 times daily; 2 to 3 cups of cold infusion or standard infusion/tisane daily; apply infused oil as needed topically.

Uses: Goldenrod grows prolifically in my area. I gather it in copious amounts every year because it has so many important uses. Goldenrod has received a bad rap because it's confused with ragweed. Ragweed is a completely different plant. The two do not even look alike, but goldenrod is in full bloom when ragweed allergies hit.

Many people have mistakenly cursed this plant, believing it to be the cause of their allergy symptoms, often called hay fever. In fact, goldenrod is an effective remedy against serious allergenic rhinitis (inflammation of the mucous membranes in the nose), including hay fever.

Goldenrod is probably known best for its benefits for urinary tract infections, bladder infections, and kidney problems of all sorts. Goldenrod is trophorestorative to the kidneys. If I were in the position of caring for someone with swollen feet and low back pain, without any other symptoms and having no tests available, goldenrod would likely be part of my treatment plan.

Goldenrod makes a wonderful addition to salves and massage creams. It soothes and relaxes achy, sore muscles and joint pain, especially from arthritis.

Contraindications: No known contraindications.

❦ GRINDELIA
Grindelia robusta, G. squarrosa

Parts Used: Flowers, leaves.

Actions: Antipruritic, expectorant, sedative.

Preparations: Dried tincture (1:5 in 95% alcohol).

Dose: 30 to 60 drops of tincture, 3 or 4 times daily.

Uses: As far as I know, grindelia does only a few things, but it does those few things exceptionally well. Grindelia is an efficient expectorant used for whooping cough, asthma, emphysema, and chronic bronchitis. It is better suited for the ongoing prevention of asthma, as opposed to an asthma attack.

Grindelia is also a great remedy for all sorts of itchy annoyances, including poison ivy, poison oak, bug bites, and stings. Jewel weed (impatiens) is often given as a remedy for poison ivy and poison oak, but if I don't have that, grindelia is a great alternative, especially made into a spray with plantain and calendula vinegars.

According to British herbalist and author Maud Grieve, grindelia has an action similar to atropine, a drug given to stabilize the heart rate after a heart attack and during surgery (it dries up body fluids to prevent choking on saliva during surgery).

I have never been in the position of having to administer grindelia to someone who just had a heart attack. However, after some digging, I was able to find that G. squarrosa was listed in *The British Pharmaceutical Codex* in 1911 as having an atropine-like effect on the heart.

Contraindications: If taken in larger-than-recommended dosages, grindelia might be irritating to people with kidney or gastrointestinal problems.

❧ HAWTHORN
Cragtaegus spp.

Parts Used: Fresh or dried berries, flowers, and leaves.

Actions: Antiarrhythmic, antioxidant, cardioprotective, cardiotonic, hypotensive.

Preparations: Fresh tincture from leaves or flowers (1:2 in 75% alcohol); dried tincture from leaves, flowers, or berries (1:5 in 50% alcohol); tisane from fresh or dried leaves or flowers; decoction from fresh or dried berries.

Dose: 30 to 60 drops of tincture, 3 to 6 times daily; 2 to 3 cups of tisane or decoction, 3 to 4 times daily.

Uses: Hawthorn is a well-researched herb known for its heart health properties. The leaves, flowers, and berries contain oligomeric procyanidins (OPCs) and flavonoids, both of which have antioxidant effects. The leaves have more OPCs, while the flowers and berries have more flavonoids. This antioxidant content helps to inhibit oxidation and degradation of cells.

Hawthorn is a mild hypotensive. If you were using hawthorn for high blood pressure, and you didn't see improvement, you would most likely need a larger dose, an additional dose, or perhaps both.

What hawthorn is most known for is its protective actions on the heart. Hawthorn is used to stabilize heart rhythm after a heart attack, as well as to heal the heart from the damage of a heart attack. Hawthorn is also used to improve the strength of heart beats.

Hawthorn has been well researched in several double-blind, randomized, placebo-controlled studies that clearly demonstrate its safety and effectiveness, even when individuals were also taking a number of powerful prescription cardiac medications. In some cases, hawthorn was used by itself, and in others combined with additional herbs such as passionflower. In still more studies, hawthorn was combined with nutritional support from coenzyme Q10 and magnesium.

Contraindications: Use caution if taking other cardiac medication, or medication to lower blood pressure. No known contraindications for pregnancy and breastfeeding.

⚘ HYSSOP
Hyssopus officinalis

Parts Used: Leaves, flowers.

Actions: Antirheumatic, diaphoretic, emmenagogue, expectorant, stimulant.

Preparations: Fresh tincture (1:2 in 95% alcohol); dried tincture (1:5 in 75% alcohol); tisane; syrup.

Dose: 30 to 60 drops of tincture, 3 or 4 times daily; 2 to 3 cups of tisane daily; 1 teaspoon of syrup every 2 hours as needed.

Uses: If there were only one herb that I could have for chest congestion or a feeling of tightness in the chest, I would pick hyssop. Hyssop opens "stuck" conditions. If you feel as if a pending infection is "gripping" at your chest, or if your chest and head feel like a solid mass that isn't budging, my top pick for you is hyssop.

I take hyssop in a tea blend at the first sign of an infection (see Respiratory Infection Tea on page 150). Often, I don't end up getting sick. Of course, getting that run down, "I'm starting to get a cold" feeling is a sign to rest. Trying to rest and not being able to do so because of congestion and chills is beyond frustrating. But if you don't rest, you can be sure that the infection will catch up with you eventually. Hyssop can help you get the rest you need, by clearing the lungs and warming up the body.

Hyssop is often combined with horehound in syrups made with honey. I like to combine hyssop with clove for a different yet pleasant taste combination and for synergism. As good as hyssop is, it works much better when clove is added. Most studies on clove focus on essential oil of clove, a valuable natural medicine. Thankfully, cloves are high in essential oil content, and the oil has been shown to be highly antimicrobial, warming, and analgesic. I have found clove's analgesic properties are pronounced in a tea or decoction.

Although hyssop is best known for providing respiratory relief, it is also effective as a topical analgesic and bruise treatment. Consumed as a tisane, hyssop is a remedy for rheumatism and arthritic conditions. In keeping with releasing "stuck" conditions, a woman who tends to skip menstrual cycles or has late or delayed menstruation can take hyssop as a tisane or tincture to release what physicians of a century or two ago would have called "stagnation" or "congestion" of the uterus.

Contraindications: Do not take during pregnancy.

❧ JUNIPER
Juniperus spp.

Parts Used: Berries, leaves.

Actions: Antibacterial, antifungal, antirheumatic, anti-inflammatory, antiseptic, antiviral, diuretic, emmenagogue, nephroprotective.

Preparations: Dried tincture (1:5 in 75% alcohol); decoction of berries or leaves; powder of the berries; essential oil of the berries.

Dose: 20 to 30 drops of tincture, 2 or 3 times daily; topically as a decoction to disinfect or as a steam, use as needed; as a wound powder as needed; as drops of essential oil in a nebulizing diffuser (follow diffuser's instructions on how many drops to use with your unit) or 3-5 drops in a bowl of steaming water (always use caution not to burn yourself with steam).

Uses: Juniper is a local antibiotic, excellent for urinary tract infections (UTIs), kidney complaints, and candida. It is effective against some very tough bacteria, such as E. coli, salmonella, clostridium, listeria, Helicobacter pylori, Klebsiella pneumoniae, and various staphylococcus and streptococcus strains.

Juniper has shown activity against tuberculosis, which is very fortunate for us. While many people think of tuberculosis as a disease of past centuries, it hasn't gone away. Tuberculosis has a 50% mortality rate without treatment, and strains of tuberculosis are developing drug resistance. One strain is completely resistant to all antibiotics.

In the face of drug-resistant bacteria, we need other options. Even if we do not see a global pandemic for another 100 years, and the economy is able to trudge along for another 50 years, we will face a crisis over antibiotic resistance in our lifetimes. Juniper, and other antibiotic herbs, offer an alternative to ineffective antibiotics.

The berries are best for UTIs, which often are caused by E. coli, as well as kidney infections. The overuse of juniper essential oil in extremely high concentrations could irritate the kidneys. Such misuse is not easy to do, and therefore easily avoided. Berries and leaves can both be used, individually or together, as a steam for respiratory infections, as can the essential oil.

All parts of the plant can be boiled and decocted for use as a disinfectant, which can be used much like modern hand sanitizer. Use it to wipe down counters and as a spray disinfectant on doorknobs and medical instruments. Juniper essential oil can be added to the wash water for laundry from a "sick room," or to a salve or gel for sanitation, but its best purpose is in a nebulizing diffuser for respiratory infections. You can also add essential oil to salves and lotions for massaging into sore muscles and joints.

As an antiviral, Juniper has shown activity against SARS and is an appropriate place to start in treating a person with a coronavirus similar to SARS like MERS, which was found to have been transmitted to humans from camels. We may someday be faced with different previously unknown zoonotic viruses, and in coming up with treatments for diseases we have never heard of, a good starting place will be to know what has worked for similar viruses in the past.

Contraindications: Because Juniper is an emmenagogue, it is best avoided in pregnancy. Long-term, internal use of juniper is not recommended. Thankfully, most of juniper's uses are short-term, such as for a UTI or a respiratory infection. If using it for tuberculosis, be mindful that juniper is similar to oil of turpentine and can be toxic with frequent, ongoing use. A sign of toxicity is urine that smells like violets. If that happens, stop use immediately. Tuberculosis requires treatment from 6 months to 1 year, so be sure to have other herbal antibiotics on hand in case toxins build up.

❧ LAVENDER
Lavendula angustifolia, L. vera

Parts Used: Flowers.

Actions: Analgesic, antibacterial, antiviral, antifungal, decongestant, diaphoretic, hypotensive, nervine, sedative, vulnerary.

Preparations: Tisane; infused oil; essential oil; hydrosol.

Dose: As needed.

Uses: The use of lavender flowers in teas, infused oils, and powders has largely been overshadowed by the use of lavender essential oil in most blog articles aimed at DIYers and homesteading types due to heavy marketing from essential oil companies. However, whole lavender flowers are a versatile ingredient in herbal preparations. Lavender tea, just lavender or in a blend with other calming herbs, is desirable for inducing a sense of calm. A strong infusion can also be used to wash surfaces (but not to disinfect on its own; use the essential oil instead), and bundles in potpourri will scent a room. Lavender is often used to scent medicinal herbal formulas that might otherwise be unpleasant to smell.

Lavender's aromatic flowers are used in eye and neck pillows, herbal steams, and herbal baths. Wrap sprigs of lavender flowers in a muslin bag or cheesecloth so you don't have to fish the petals out of the tub afterward. Lavender infused steam is excellent for relaxation and the respiratory system.

Lavender essential oil is very widely used. Lavender essential oil is so popular that it is often adulterated in some way. France exports more lavender essential oil each year than it produces, which should say something about how often it is faked.

The popularity of lavender oil is well deserved. Use the oil for disinfecting surfaces and scenting laundry. Lavender steam, either from the oil or the flowers, is a mild, gentle decongestant. Applied to the temples, the essential oil can help relieve a stress headache.

Lavender essential oil is quite possibly my favorite remedy for earache pain. A drop or two on a cotton ball, shaped into an earplug, and the pain (and infection) goes away. It's nice to insert the cotton ball earplug, and then place a hot water bottle with enough layers of towel in between the water bottle and the ear to protect the skin in case the bottle is too hot. The heat and the lavender essential oil work like magic.

Lavender and lavender essential oil are used in various personal care products including soaps, lotions, and salves. The essential oil is often used in formulations to promote the healing of burned skin.

Contraindications: No known contraindications. However, use caution with lavender essential oil. Essential oils are not to be ingested. While lavender oil can often be used on the skin undiluted (without a carrier oil, like grapeseed oil), not everyone's skin will react the same way.

ℋ LEMON BALM
Melissa officinalis

Parts Used: Fresh or dried flowers and leaves.

Actions: Antiviral, anxiolytic, carminative, diaphoretic, febrifuge, nervine, sedative.

Preparations: Fresh tincture (1:2 in 95% alcohol); dried tincture (1:5 in 75% alcohol); tisane.

Dose: 30 to 60 drops of tincture, 3 or 4 times daily; 2 to 3 cups of tisane daily.

Uses: Lemon balm is used primarily as a gentle calming herb and mild sedative to ease away tension. Its pleasant flavor can make "medicinal-tasting" herbs more palatable. This is especially important for young children, who often refuse anything that doesn't taste good to their yet-to-develop palates.

This plant is safe to use in herbal blends for pregnant women dealing with nausea, heartburn, and nervousness.

Lemon balm can help bring down a fever by inducing sweating. Sweating is one way the body can purge itself of waste and detoxify itself. Sweat also cools the skin, which helps to relieve a fever.

There are many good, solid, mainstream studies that support the normalcy and even the need for fever when ill. Fever is an important function in fighting off an infection. Fever is uncomfortable, but it's a natural self-defense mechanism against illness. However, if you have to bring a fever down, doing so with a sudorific at least assists with the normal function of the body (sweating, waste removal) instead of just blocking a response to illness.

Lemon balm has one more specific use: as a remedy for herpes sores. Apply the tincture, tisane, infused oil, or salve directly to the sores.

Contraindications: No known contraindications.

✻ LICORICE
Glycerrhiza glabra

Parts Used: Root.

Actions: Antiviral, demulcent, estrogenic, expectorant, immunostimulant, synergistic.

Preparations: Dried tincture (1:5 in 20% alcohol, 60% water, and 20% vinegar); cold infusion; decoction; syrup.

Dose: Use tincture in blends with other herbs as a synergist or to add antiviral actions; 2 to 3 cups of decoction or infusion (with other herbs) daily; 1 teaspoon of syrup every 2 hours as needed.

Uses: Licorice tastes good, is a soothing demulcent, and is effective against a range of viruses. As a demulcent, licorice encourages the body to lubricate the mucosa, protecting it and improving immune response.

Licorice is also a potent synergist. Caution is called for when taking licorice while on medication, as the licorice may increase the effects of the medication. Licorice may also increase the effects of other herbs, but this can be a benefit when blending cold and flu remedies.

Licorice is often considered an estrogenic herb. It does not contain estrogen, but it has been found to increase the effects of estrogen. To what extent is up for debate. Licorice has been blamed for causing male breast tissue to grow. However, licorice also addresses most of the symptoms associated with polycystic ovarian syndrome (PCOS). This leads me to question if licorice is really increasing estrogen or lowering testosterone. In either case, the estrogenic effects will last for a few weeks after licorice use stops.

It's best to take licorice in small amounts and to be sure to get enough potassium. At high doses, licorice can sometimes cause an increase in blood pressure. Keeping licorice doses within the recommended levels and getting enough potassium should prevent this problem. If elevated blood pressure has been an issue, check your blood pressure regularly while using licorice—or skip licorice altogether.

Although licorice comes with a few cautions, it is very antiviral and a great choice for any respiratory infection. It is effective against influenza, SARS, West Nile virus, hepatitis, chicken pox, and measles. It is also a very safe herb to take as long as you keep the various warnings in mind.

Contraindications: Not for use during pregnancy. Do not use with uncontrolled hypertension. Use caution if taking medications.

❦ LOBELIA
Lobelia inflata

Parts Used: Entire plant.

Actions: Antispasmodic, emetic, expectorant.

Preparations: Fresh tincture (1:4 in 75% alcohol and 25% apple cider vinegar); dried acetum (1:7 in 100% apple cider vinegar); infused oil.

Dose: Low-dose herb, 5 to 20 drops of fresh or dried extract, up to 4 times daily. Begin with the absolute lowest dose, adjust upward with control and only as needed; take as tisane by the cupful as needed to induce vomiting (tincture is not emetic).

Uses: Lobelia is a powerful herb. It is a supreme antispasmodic and top-notch expectorant. This is one of a couple of herbs capable of addressing an acute asthma attack.

There is no better herb for bringing a muscle out of contraction. Lobelia can even relax muscles in someone suffering from lockjaw. However, this comes with some risk. The heart is a muscle, and it is affected by muscle relaxers like lobelia. If you take too much lobelia, or if you already have a weak heart, you may inadvertently stop the heart. With a little attention to the dosage, however, lobelia can be a safe and effective remedy for serious spasms, asthma, and even as a first response to anaphylaxis (to be followed up with an antihistamine, such as ample doses of nettle tincture and tea).

Staying within the safe range and always trying to stay at the lower end of the dosage recommendations is a smart idea, especially when treating asthma. Naturally, a lot depends on the person with asthma. Use with caution and common sense. The biggest risk, as I see it, is lack of experience with this herb and, as a result, becoming nervous during an emergency and using too much.

Lobelia is an emetic herb. If you take too much, it will make you vomit. I have had lobelia as both tea and tincture, and I did not become ill. It does not have an immediate emetic response, such as happens with ipecac. Lobelia could be included in a tea as an expectorant in combination with better tasting respiratory herbs, as it is not the most pleasant tasting of herbs.

Although lobelia should not be used during pregnancy because of its emetic nature, it can be helpful when a miscarriage threatens. It is an antispasmodic, and the rationale for using it in this situation is that it will get the uterus to stop contracting. It is most often used in combination with other herbal tinctures for this purpose.

Lobelia can also be infused in oil and used either as a massage oil or as an ingredient in salves and lotions. This can be very useful when dealing with jaw clenching, TMJ problems, and trying to reduce (to return to proper position) a misaligned jaw gently with manual techniques.

Contraindications: Use lobelia with great caution. Anyone with a weak heart or cardiac problems should not use it. Avoid use in someone who is sleepy, depressed, or using alcohol. Not for use during pregnancy, except when appropriate to prevent miscarriage.

❦ MA HUANG
Ephedra sinica, E. vulgaris

Parts Used: Stems.

Actions: Analgesic, antispasmodic, decongestant, expectorant, stimulant.

Preparations: Dried tincture (1:5 in 60% alcohol, 30% water, 10% apple cider vinegar); decoction.

Dose: 10 to 30 drops of tincture, 1 to 3 times daily; 2 to 3 cups of decoction daily.

Uses: Ma huang, or better known in the United States as ephedra, is banned from sale. You can, however, order the seeds, grow it, and make your own tincture. You just cannot sell it. Unfortunately, ephedra was being marketed as a weight loss product. And, if one pill is good, then lots of pills must be better, right? Because of this misuse, the FDA banned ephedra from being sold in any product.

Ephedra has been used as an expectorant, pain reliever, appetite suppressant, and stimulant. People taking ephedra need to be careful not to take too much. It can raise blood pressure, cause irregular heart beats, and reduce appetite. Ultimately, taking too much could lead to heart attack or coma.

I have seen the hot tea of ephedra stop an asthma attack: 10 drops of tincture were given immediately while the tea was brewing. Then the person having the attack was able to sip the tea until the entire event was over. Hot beverages, including hot coffee, can help with an asthma attack in a pinch as well.

Since I don't have anyone with asthma in my house, and there are other herbs that work wonderfully for respiratory complaints and muscle spasms, I recently started carrying ephedra tincture in my emergency kit for a totally different reason—as a type of emergency herbal EpiPen, but with a much longer shelf life than the EpiPen.

We keep bees. We keep them for honey, wax, propolis, barter value, food value, and general medicinal value. None of us are allergic to bee stings at the moment. But this is always in the back of my mind: What if one of us developed an allergy to bee stings, and there was no medical help? What would we do?

Allergies to bee stings, like allergies to certain foods, can cause the body to go into anaphylaxis. This in an incredibly serious situation that could easily result in death if not treated. What is a prepper to do if he or she, or a loved one, starts to go into anaphylaxis?

The active ingredient in an EpiPen is epinephrine. Epinephrine and ephedrine (an alkaloid in ephedra) have very similar actions. However, ephedrine isn't as fast acting or as strong as epinephrine. It is an option, however, when no other option exists.

The key to taking ephedra safely is not overdoing the dosage out of nervousness. I would start out giving the lowest dose, in this case 10 drops of tincture. I would then give 60 drops of nettle tincture. The epinephrine in an EpiPen is merely a stop-gag measure to buy time to get the anaphylaxis patient to a hospital. Once at the hospital, the patient would be given a strong dose of antihistamine medication, such as Benadryl. When antihistamine medications are not available, the antihistamine properties of nettle would be an alternative. I would repeat both the ephedra and nettle tinctures every 15 minutes for an hour, and then reassess. It may be a good idea to know how to insert a nasal trumpet for intubation to keep airway passages open in case the herbs do not work fast enough. (Even the pharmaceutical EpiPen and Benadryl may not work quickly enough, and intubation is necessary.)

Ephedra has a somewhat less potent cousin in the United States called Mormon tea (E. viridis). In fact, there are many varieties throughout the country. Find out which one grows near you.

Contraindications: Do not take when pregnant. Not for anyone with high blood pressure or with cardiac arrhythmia or other heart problems.

❧ MARSHMALLOW
Althaea officinalis

Parts Used: Roots, leaves.

Actions: Antibacterial, anti-inflammatory, demulcent, expectorant, hypoglycemic.

Preparations: Cold infusion from dried roots (preferable) or standard infusion of leaves; cold infusion can be used as syrup base.

Dose: Take cold infusion as needed, preferably warmed up, for coughs or any respiratory complaint; take the cold infusion 3 to 6 cups per day as part of UTI care to soothe tissues until symptoms go away; apply topically as needed to assist in wound healing, especially for burn care.

Uses: Marshmallow is a mucilaginous, demulcent herb. This slippery, slick herb creates a thick liquid that coats, soothes, and encourages the body to hydrate the mucosa. This way, even if the marshmallow doesn't come in direct contact with the mucosa, it still has a lubricating effect on it.

This soothing action helps to quell inflammation, especially of a sore throat, while also encouraging productive coughing. Marshmallow is appropriate for bronchitis and whooping cough in addition to sore throats. And while it does wonders for the respiratory system, it also helps soothe inflamed and delicate tissues from urinary tract infections.

Although both the roots and leaves are usable, I far prefer the roots. Skip any thoughts of tincturing this herb. The results can very easily turn gloppy. Sometimes I brew the leaves like regular tea, but I'm much more partial to the roots as a cold infusion.

Marshmallow is loaded with pectin, which helps create a soothing, thick, calming, gel-like liquid. I like to add this thickened, gelatinous cold infusion instead of honey for syrups for diabetics who need to avoid excess sugar. It will be a runny syrup, as marshmallow cold infusion is not as viscous as honey, and the shelf life will be significantly decreased (3 days in refrigerator) without the honey. But, when extra sugar must be avoided, this is a good choice.

Making a cold infusion is very easy. Just put 1 cup of dry herbs into a quart mason jar, and fill to the top with room-temperature water. Screw the lid on, and wait at least 4 hours (I prefer overnight). After 4 hours, you will have a usable cold infusion. This cold infusion extracts the polysaccharides without all the starches. The strained liquid will be golden in color.

The cold infusion is helpful to anyone with a gastrointestinal problem. If you are working on healing your gut, you will want to check out this herb. Marshmallow, on occasion, can lower blood sugar, but only mildly so. Be aware if you take antidiabetic medication, check your blood sugar, and marshmallow should pose no problem.

Contraindications: No known contraindications.

❦ MILK THISTLE
Silybum marianum

Parts Used: Seeds.

Actions: Bitter, cholagogue, depurative, estrogenic, galactagogue.

Preparations: Ground seeds; tincture (1:3 in 95% alcohol).

Dose: 30 to 60 drops of tincture, 3 or 4 times daily; ground seeds by the tablespoon 2 to 3 times daily

Uses: Milk thistle helps support and regenerate liver cells. It is a bitter tonic, and the most important herb to consider when the liver is diseased. This is the first herb I would include in a plan for someone with cirrhosis of the liver.

Milk thistle has many of the same properties as dandelion. There are differences, however. Although wonderful at improving liver function, milk thistle has some estrogen-like actions, making it a potential herbal helper to women going through menopause. On the other hand, if you have a hormonal imbalance with too much estrogen, like PCOS, use of milk thistle for liver support should be short-term use only, maybe 3 weeks to 3 months, and not on an ongoing basis. However, dandelion does not have the cell regeneration properties of milk thistle. Dandelion won't increase lactation.

Contraindications: It is unknown if milk thistle's estrogen-like actions impact estrogen-sensitive cancers or other estrogen-related complications. Considering that dandelion has many of the same properties as milk thistle, I would use dandelion instead.

❦ MOTHERWORT
Leonurus cardiaca, L. sibericus

Parts Used: Leaves, flowers.

Actions: Antispasmodic, anxiolytic, cardiac tonic, diaphoretic, diuretic, emmenagogue, nervine.

Preparations: Fresh tincture (1:2 in 95% alcohol); dried tincture (1:5 in 60% alcohol); tisane; syrup.

Dose: 30 to 40 drops of tincture, 3 or 4 times daily; 2 to 3 cups of tisane daily; 1 tablespoon of syrup, 4 or 5 times daily.

Uses: Motherwort is calming and stabilizing, just as you would expect a "mother" to be. Motherwort exerts its influence on the heart and the thyroid, as well as on menstruation, cramping, menopausal hot flashes, and afterbirth healing.

This herb is associated with a happy heart, both emotionally and physically. Good for anyone who has suffered great loss, motherwort can help lift the feeling of darkness that sometimes comes with experiencing trauma. It is appropriate for anyone experiencing mood swings, especially hormonal mood swings.

Motherwort has a long history of use to relieve premenstrual symptoms and to bring on delayed menses. It relaxes smooth muscle tissue, thus helping to calm cramping. Stress and stress hormones are a frequent factor in irregular menstrual cycles, and could be a significant issue after a disaster.

Also consider motherwort's impressive cardiac benefits. The herb is useful in slowing a too-rapid heart rate and in establishing a steady rhythm in people with arrhythmia.

Contraindications: I have read warnings against using motherwort on anyone who has hypothyroid issues (underactive thyroid). However, my observations do not support this warning, nor have I seen any published studies to support this warning either.

❦ MULLEIN
Verbascum thapsus

Parts Used: Fresh or dried flowers; dried leaves (from first year plants only).

Actions: Analgesic, antibacterial, anti-inflammatory, astringent, demulcent, emollient, expectorant, sedative (mild).

Preparations: Infused oil from flowers; tisane from leaves.

Dose: Topically as needed; 2 to 3 cups of tisane daily.

Uses: One of the better known traditional remedies is mullein infused oil. Typically, the flowers are infused in olive oil to make a pain-relieving, anti-inflammatory, antibacterial remedy for ear infections. The infused oil can be added to salves and lotions to treat a range of conditions including dry skin, burns, scrapes, and arthritic joints.

Mullein leaves are used for respiratory complaints and diarrhea. The leaves are both astringent and demulcent, which makes for an ideal, if mild, diarrhea remedy. I add it to other astringent herbs when the diarrhea is severe.

For respiratory complaints, mullein can be made into a tea. The only issue is that mullein is quite fluffy and bulky, even when dried. It can take up a lot of space, making it challenging to get enough herb into the blend and still have it covered by the water.

The leaves take a long time to dry. They are large and soft, and would make an ideal substitute for toilet paper. Pick leaves only after the sun has risen and burned away any morning dew. When preparing mullein for storage in your dried medicinal herb collection, cut or tear the leaf along the vein to the stem. I don't generally dry my herbs in a dehydrator, but for mullein, it's a major help. Chop the leaves into small pieces, and use your dehydrator on the lowest setting.

When you think the leaves are completely dry, run a knife through them to chop them again and put them back in the dehydrator for another hour or two. Use a fruit roll sheet in your dehydrator if necessary. If you do not have a dehydrator, dry the leaves in the oven on the lowest setting. Give them lots of air and room on the tray.

Contraindications: No known contraindications.

❧ NETTLE
Urtica dioica

Parts Used: Young leaves, root, seeds.

Actions: Analgesic, anti-edema, astringent, diuretic, hypotensive, renal trophorestorative, tonic.

Preparations: Tincture from fresh leaves, roots, or new seeds (1:2 in 95% alcohol); tincture from dried leaves, roots, or older seeds (1:5 in 50% alcohol); tisane of dried or fresh leaves; syrup of dried or fresh leaves.

Dose: Use 30 to 60 drops of leaf (fresh or dried) tincture as antihistamine for more serious allergic reactions, 3 to 4 cups of tisane (fresh or dried leaves) to relieve swelling, release excess fluids, and for minor allergic reactions. Use 30 to 60 drops of fresh or dried root tincture, 3 to 4 times per day for prostate health and male pattern baldness. Use tisane or an acetum of the leaves and/or roots, fresh or dried, as a nourishing hair rinse. Use 20 to 40 drops of tincture made with older seeds for adrenal support and as a mood-enhancing adaptogen. Use 60 drops of tincture from new nettle seeds 3 times daily for serious kidney illness.

Uses: Nettle is an overlooked superfood. While an exotic ingredient that exploits some native population in a far-flung corner of the globe is hyped as the latest and greatest find, we ignore one of the most nutritious plants growing almost everywhere in the United States.

Nettle is often used to relieve edema, joint pain, and allergies. However, the applications for nettle are far more than I can list here. So much of our health is tied to nutrition, and nettle is a nutritional treasure trove high in iron, calcium, potassium, and chlorophyll. There is an expanded section on nutrition and uses for nettle in Chapter 6.

Chlorophyll is used as an "internal cleanser" or "blood cleanser." The fact that chlorophyll-rich nettle significantly helps to cut down on body odor may be the origin of such claims.

Nettle does sting if not handled properly. Nettle stings were used medicinally from at least as early as the Middle Ages. The nettle stalk was wielded like a whip across the suffering part of the body. This brought the sting (and therefore the medicine) to the site of pain. It was used mainly for arthritis conditions.

Nettle, specifically nettle root, has important benefits for men. Nettle root (best taken as a tincture for this issue) helps relieve prostate symptoms. When combined with saw palmetto, nettle tincture may also be a treatment for male pattern baldness.[8]

Nettle is known for supporting the kidneys and adrenal glands. Nettle seeds share these traits along with the leaves. Nettle seeds have an adaptogenic effect, bringing the body back into balance, and instilling a sense of well-being. The fresh, newly harvested seeds, however, when made into a tincture appear to be trophorestorative to the kidneys. If I

---

8   A study published by the American Botanical Counsel, "Saw Palmetto, Nettles, and Pygeum for Male Pattern Baldness" showed nettle, when combined with saw palmetto, to be an effective and safe approach to male pattern baldness. Karen Dean, "Saw Palmetto, Nettles, and Pygeum for male pattern baldness," *American Botanical Counsel* 49 (September 2000): 31.

had to deal with serious kidney disease without the benefit of modern medicine, I would include tincture of fresh nettle seeds in my plan.[9]

Any survivalists worth their salt will want to have nettle in their area, and know how to harvest it and how to prepare it. Consume nettle cooked, not raw (cooking removes the sting). Use it as you would any dark, leafy green in soups or steamed. The stalk can be made into fiber for spinning or into cordage.

Contraindications: No known contraindications. Do not overuse nettle. It can be very drying. Overuse of nettle can result in a condition known as uticaria (hives). If this happens, stop using nettle, and rub crushed dock leaves (any kind of dock such as yellow dock or burdock) on the hives. Or if you have baking soda, make a paste and rub it on the hives.

❧ OATS
Avena sativa

Parts Used: Milky oat tops, oatstraw.

Actions: Anti-inflammatory, antispasmodic, demulcent, emollient, nervine, sedative (mild), tonic.

Preparations: Gruel (oatmeal); tisane.

Dose: As needed.

Uses: If you have ever wondered why oatmeal is such a comfort food, it's because it really does make you feel better. Oats are a calming nervine that takes the edge off any stressful day. It is also useful when your skin feels too dry.

Oats have countless uses in skin care products, including soaps. It can relieve itchy, dry skin associated with eczema and psoriasis, and itches from sunburns and chickenpox, as well as menopausal dryness.

---

9   In an article, "Urtica Semen Reduces Serum Creatinine Levels" by Jonathon Treasure, he details the benefits of nettle seed for serious kidney disease. Jonathon Treasure, "Urtica Semen Reduces Serum Creatinine Levels," *Journal of the American Herbalist Guild* 4 (2003): 22–25.

If you are suffering from insomnia, try a bowl of oatmeal or a cup of tea made from the immature tops or oatstraw a half hour before going to bed.

Contraindications: No known contraindications. If you are sensitive to gluten, be sure to get oats processed in a gluten-free facility for your long-term food storage.

❦ PEPPERMINT
Mentha × piperita

Parts Used: Leaves harvested before the plant flowers.

Actions: Analgesic, anti-emetic, anti-inflammatory, antispasmodic, cardiotonic, carminative, decongestant, diaphoretic, refrigerant.

Preparations: Tisane; essential oil; hydrosol.

Dose: As needed.

Uses: Peppermint is high in aromatic, volatile oils, making it a viable option for those who want to distill their own essential oils. Peppermint can grow almost anywhere, and to the chagrin of many gardeners, it does. But the addition of well-rotted manure and moisture make peppermint crops for essential oil distillation a much more profitable venture.

Peppermint is the source of one of the most versatile essential oils. Because of the high concentration of menthol, peppermint oil makes a good pain reliever. Add it to salves and lotions for sore muscles. It is a great addition to creams for tired feet and is a favorite in soaps.

In a diffuser, peppermint essential oil is a powerful decongestant. Applied in drops to the temples, it can stop a migraine in its tracks. It has saved me from many lost days due to migraines. However, it must be applied immediately at the first signs of a migraine. It will still help somewhat if the migraine is already well entrenched. But if taken right at the very start, peppermint essential oil often can prevent the migraine from happening in the first place.

The oil can be used diluted in a spray to disinfect surfaces and repel pests, especially mice and ants. (This is very helpful when you have a cabin in the woods.) The oil can freshen up and disinfect a sick room.

Peppermint tea thins out mucous secretions, making it a useful decongestant for both upper and lower respiratory infections. Because it tastes so pleasant, peppermint is an easy medicine to give to children or use in blends to improve the taste of other herbs.

This aromatic herb is also a carminative and calms nausea. It is useful in alleviating morning sickness. Peppermint can also help to calm colon spasms.

The hydrosol is cooling. It can be used to spray on a burn, or on the forehead and neck of someone with a fever as a comfort measure.

Contraindications: No known contraindications.

❧ PLANTAIN
Plantago major, P. lanceolata

Parts Used: Leaves, seeds.

Actions: Astringent, demulcent, depurative, laxative, refrigerant, styptic, vulnerary.

Preparations: Fresh tincture (1:2 in 95% alcohol); dried tincture (1:5 in 50%); cold infusion; standard infusion; decoction of seeds; poultice.

Dose: 30 to 60 drops of tincture, 3 or 4 times daily; 3 to 4 cups of leaf infusion or seed decoction daily; topically as a poultice as needed.

Uses: Plantain is one of those great medicines right under our noses. It's in nearly every lawn. I'm sure my neighbors are irritated that our lawn is loaded with plantain and dandelions every year. All I see is beautiful, free, natural medicine. Obviously, spraying the lawn is out of the question.

Plantain contains a very soothing, cooling, and demulcent inner juice. It is ideal for burns, bites, cuts, and scrapes. However, when it come to caring for burns, do not waste time harvesting leaves from the lawn to mash up and apply to the burn. The first rule of burn care is to stop the damage from spreading.

Unless you have copious amounts of plantain juice on hand, you're better off cooling the burn with clean water. Once the burn has been brought under control, then you can apply plantain in a poultice to the burn. It will work wonders then.

Plantain tincture can be used as a styptic, as well as for bringing down a fever.

This herb is a good ingredient in drawing, blister, and wound care salves. The leaves are highly astringent, which makes plantain excellent for skin healing as well as diarrhea. However, plantain seeds can be used as a laxative.

Contraindications: No known contraindications.

❧ SAGE
Salvia officinalis

Parts Used: Leaves.

Actions: Astringent, antibacterial, antifungal, antiperspirant, estrogenic, emmenagogue, stimulant.

Preparations: Fresh tincture (1:2 in 95% alcohol); dried tincture (1:5 in 75% alcohol); tisane; syrup; essential oil.

Dose: 30 to 60 drops of tincture, 3 or 4 times daily; 2 to 3 cups of tisane daily; syrup as needed; essential oil 3 to 6 drops for steam inhalation, or the number of drops indicated by your aromatherapy diffuser, or topically in a carrier oil (dilution rate is 6 drops of essential oil diluted in 1 ounce of carrier oil).

Uses: Sage is an aromatic and culinary herb with some very interesting properties. Unlike the other estrogenic herbs, like milk thistle and licorice, sage actually does contain phytoestrogens, and doesn't just mimic estrogen. This along with sage's astringent quality makes the plant a good option for women dealing with menopausal night sweats. Night sweats are unpleasant enough in a world with air conditioning, but in a post-disaster world they will be miserable for both parties attempting to sleep in a soaked bed.

Sage is antibacterial and makes for an effective mouthwash. It is taken as a tea to bring on delayed menstruation. The aroma of sage is used to help improve both focus and memory. The essential oil can also be used for delayed menstruation diluted in a carrier oil and massaged onto the abdomen. Sage essential oil diluted in coconut oil can be applied to the scalp to fight dandruff, or anywhere on the skin to fight fungal infections.

Even though sage can be quite drying, it makes an excellent cough syrup in combination with a other herbs such as horehound, anise hyssop, elecompane, mullein, and marshmallow.

Contraindications: Not for use during pregnancy.

❧ ST. JOHN'S WORT
Hypericum perforatum

Parts Used: Flowers, leaves.

Actions: Analgesic, anxiolytic, astringent, cell proliferator, expectorant, nervine, vulnerary.

Preparations: Fresh tincture (1:2 in 95% alcohol); dried tincture (1:5 in 75% alcohol); infused oil from fresh plant parts; capsules from dried plant parts; tisane from dried plant parts; infused honey.

Dose: 30 to 40 drops of tincture, 3 or 4 times daily for relief from depression and anxiety; 2 to 3 cups of tisane daily as an expectorant; topically in infused oil over closed wounds with resulting in nerve pain; topically in infused honey for burns and open wound care as needed; capsules vary by capsule size, and either a size 0 or 1 would be appropriate.

Uses: St. John's wort is known mostly for its mood-enhancing effects for people with mild to moderate depression. While I don't mean to diminish those properties, as I think they will be lifesavers to some people, it's the wound care properties that preppers really should pay attention to. Still, keep some on hand as after a disaster, people will need anti-depressants, and there won't be help from the pharmacy.

Comfrey usually comes to mind when thinking of wounds and cell regeneration. Few remedies knit tissue back together as well as comfrey. However, comfrey has a major drawback. It is so effective that often it closes the surface of a wound too soon, leaving an unhealed wound under the surface. This is a recipe for infection. Without professional medical care available, an infection could easily become life-threatening.

St. John's wort, however, has a different habit. It heals from the inside out. This is exactly how you want a wound to heal. The challenge is, how do you get this medicine into a deep wound?

You could use a tincture, but the alcohol would not be comfortable. Also, if the wound were big, a tincture consisting of only few drops would not cover a large area. My solution is to infuse St. John's wort flowers in honey. Honey is an ideal remedy for wounds, and infusing St. John's wort flowers makes a uniquely suited wound care medicine.

An alternative is to make an infused oil of the flowers. Then add the infused oil to honey with a tiny bit of heat and a lot of elbow grease. St. John's wort is a must to include with any remedy dealing with nerve pain. The infused oil is good for making salves. St. John's wort infused oil and cayenne infused oil make an excellent salve for nerve pain. Other pain salve combinations for St. John's wort could include the infused oils of arnica, lobelia, peppermint, and white willow bark.

Contraindications: St. John's wort has a very long list of contraindications with medications, especially with other mood-enhancing pharmaceuticals. If you are taking prescription medications, it may be best to skip St. John's wort.

❧ SIDA
Sida acuta, S. cordifolia, S. rhombifolia, S. spinosa

Parts Used: Aerial parts.

Actions: Antiamoebic, antibacterial, anti-inflammatory, anti-fertility, antimalarial, antimicrobial, antiprotozoal, antivenom, antiviral, demulcent, emollient, expectorant, hematoprotectant, hypoglycemic.

Preparations: Dried tincture (1:5 in 60% alcohol), tisane (1 tablespoon apple cider vinegar or lemon juice to 6 ounces of water).

Dose: 20 to 40 drops of tincture 3 to 6 times daily; tisane 3 to 4 times daily.

Uses: Sida is a systemic antibiotic. This means it passes readily into the bloodstream and circulates around the body. Sida has been shown to be active against a range of bacteria plus some viruses. It is used to treat E. coli, salmonella, various streptococcus and staphylococcus infections, infected wounds, *Klebsiella pneumoniae,* shigella, malaria, and tuberculosis.

Sida is also a hematoprotectant, meaning that it protects the blood. One such threat from which sida has protected the blood is snake venom, specifically the venom from a South American pit viper, *Bothrops atrox.* I doubt there has been testing of sida against other venoms, but if I were bit by a pit viper and there were no doctors or functioning hospitals around, I would look for my sida tincture, and I would be taking the higher dosage at the greater frequency.

As part of the mallow family, sida is soothing and has many similar benefits as marshmallow, being emollient, expectorant, and demulcent.

Contraindications: Since the herb has been shown to stop ovulation in lab mice, it may be best to avoid it when pregnant or trying to become pregnant.

❀ SPILANTHES
Spilanthes acmella

Parts Used: Flowers, leaves, stems.

Actions: Analgesic, antifungal, anti-inflammatory, emetic.

Preparations: Fresh tincture (1:2 in 95% alcohol); dried flower buds to chew on.

Dose: By the drop on an aching tooth as needed; in a spray to spray on a sore throat as needed.

Uses: This is a relatively new herb in my repertoire, but it is absolutely impressive. Spilanthes is known as "toothache plant" for its numbing effects. If you have ever had severe mouth pain, then you know how awful it can be. Mouth pain can stop a person in his or her tracks.

Spilanthes creates a tingling, almost fizzy reaction in the mouth. It is similar to echinacea in this respect. Spilanthes tincture dropped directly on an abscess or mouth wound is a major help to anyone coping without a dentist (who may be even rarer than a doctor post-disaster). The plant can also be used to make an antibacterial mouth rinse.

Another use for spilanthes is as a remedy for ringworm. But perhaps one of the more interesting properties of spilanthes is that it can kill spirochetes (a spiral-shaped bacterium that causes Lyme disease and syphilis). Anyone who lives where Lyme disease is prevalent should grow spilanthes. Lyme is a complex disease, and it normally requires many different herbs in a comprehensive and personalized protocol. Spilanthes, however, would be in any Lyme strategy of mine.

Contraindications: No known contraindications.

⚘ THYME
Thymus vulgaris

Parts Used: Leaves.

Actions: Analgesic, antibacterial, antiviral, antifungal, antitussive, antispasmodic, expectorant.

Preparations: Fresh tincture (1:2 in 95% alcohol); dried tincture (1:5 in 75% alcohol); tisane of fresh or dried leaves; acetum of fresh or dried leaves; essential oil; syrup; infused honey.

Dose: 30 to 60 drops of tincture, 3 or 4 times daily; 2 to 3 cups of tisane daily; acetum can be taken like tincture, or added freely in foods, marinades, salad dressings, etc.; inhalation through herbal steam or with essential oil in a nebulizing diffuser as needed; syrup or infused honey as needed.

Uses: Thyme works on just about any respiratory infection, viral or bacterial. It is excellent for calming a cough and is effective against whooping cough, bronchitis, and any sore throat. Herbal steams and (the steam from) herbal baths of thyme are both effective ways to bring thyme's medicine to the respiratory system. A bath has the added benefit of using thyme to soothe the aches that often accompany a respiratory infection.

The essential oil distilled from thyme may be one of the most potent antimicrobial essential oils, if not the most potent. Thyme is certainly on my list of herbs to grow in quantity to produce some of this precious oil, which can easily be added to healing salves and used to prevent infection in cuts and scrapes.

Prepping for the unknown can be very challenging. There's no way to know for certain if it will really be enough or effective until the post-disaster situation. But we can make strong educated guesses. If there were to be an outbreak of some new and unknown contagious respiratory illness, and I had to pick just one essential oil for inhalations and disinfection, I would pick thyme. There's no guarantee that it would work, but it has a better chance than just about anything else natural that I'm aware of.

If you cannot distill your own oil, use the tincture topically on abrasions. Thyme also makes a lovely acetum.

Contraindications: As an herb, thyme doesn't have any contraindications. However, thyme essential oil does. This is a "hot" oil. It can cause great irritation to the skin, especially sensitive skin. It is not a great choice for use in a diffuser with a child, as it can be more of an irritant than a help. For children, restrict inhalation time in herbal baths and steams. Always be sure the bath or steam is not too hot. No need to risk a burn. Young children should not be left unattended in any bath, especially a relaxing one.

⅍ TURMERIC
Curcuma longa

Parts Used: Rhizome.

Actions: Analgesic, anti-cancer, anti-inflammatory, antibacterial, antifungal, cardioprotective, cholagogue, depurative, nephroprotective, neuroprotective, radioprotective, vasoprotective.

Preparations: In capsules or food. Consume with a small amount of fat and a pinch of black pepper.

Dose: Eat freely.

Uses: Turmeric is a powerhouse of an herb. It is well worth growing, although you must make some room for it in your garden, much as you would its relative ginger. Bring it in during the winter if you live in a cold climate.

A potent anti-inflammatory herb, turmeric is an herbal COX-2 inhibitor used for both osteoarthritis and rheumatoid arthritis relief. I've used turmeric and ginger together to calm inflammation.[10]

---

10   In "Chemopreventive and Therapeutic Effects of Curcumin" in *Cancer Letters*, a mini-review published by Elsiver, it is suggested that this anti-inflammatory activity is one of several reasons for turmeric's anti-carcinogenic properties. Annelyse Duvoix et al., "Chemopreventive and Therapeutic Effects of Curcumin," *Cancer Letters* 223 (2005): 181–190.

While fresh turmeric is ideal, most people have access only to the powdered form. The powder is still quite active, and may be added to foods and capsules. Turmeric is more effective if taken with some kind of fat as well as black pepper. This happens naturally in much of Indian cooking, as turmeric is a major ingredient in many curry blends. Even if you don't think you like curry, you may just not like the store-bought variety. There are plenty of recipes to test, and you'll probably find one you like.

If you aren't a curry fan, I suggest adding a pinch of black pepper and maybe washing the turmeric capsule down with dairy milk or coconut milk, or eating something with butter or coconut oil on it at about the same time. It doesn't have to be coconut oil. You could dunk some homemade bread in olive oil.

You can apply turmeric like a paste on acne, eczema, and psoriasis. Also, you can infuse turmeric in water, soak a towel in that water, and use the towel as a compress for conjunctivitis. Do be careful, as turmeric can leave a stain on skin (temporarily) and clothes (less temporarily) that may take some time to come out. Another use for turmeric is as an addition to wound powders.

Contraindications: Turmeric is not a common allergen, but rare allergic reactions have happened. Since turmeric increases bile production, it is not recommended for people with gallstones or bile duct obstruction.

❦ USNEA, A.K.A. OLD MAN'S BEARD
Usnea spp.

Parts Used: Entire lichen.

Actions: Analgesic, antibacterial, antifungal, anti-inflammatory, anti-parasitic, antiprotozoal, antiseptic, antiviral.

Preparations: Tincture and tisane, but not in the same manner all the others have been made (see below for instructions unique to usnea); wound powder.

Dose: 30 to 60 drops of tincture, 3 or 4 times daily; 2 to 3 cups of tisane daily; wound powder as needed.

Uses: Usnea is a lichen found just about everywhere. There are hundreds of species of usnea, so one likely grows in your area. Usnea makes a strong antibiotic, especially against gram-positive bacteria, including drug-resistant strains of tuberculosis.

Usnea is not a systemic antibiotic. It remains in the gastrointestinal tract, allowing it to address bacterial infections of the stomach and intestines. The powder of the dried herb is a welcome addition to wound powders.

Letting the lichen dry and then grinding it to a powder is relatively straightforward, but tincturing and tea making are less so. In his book *Herbal Antibiotics,* Stephen Harrod Buhner recommends using heat to make the tincture either in a slow cooker or in an oven on a very low setting.

Using the standard ratio for dry herbs in a menstruum of 1:5 (1 ounce of herb by weight to 5 ounces of menstruum by volume), and the menstruum being 50% alcohol and 50% water, place your dry herbs and the water portion in a slow cooker. Cover and set on warm for 48 hours. I've tried this on low, but it just got too hot in my slow cooker. I had to use the warm setting instead. Make sure the lid is on securely, so you don't lose too much moisture to evaporation.

After 48 hours, transfer the mush to a mason jar. After it has cooled but is still warm, add the alcohol portion. Put the lid on the jar, allow the mixture to macerate for 2 weeks, shake the jar once daily (or whenever you think about it), and after 2 weeks, strain out the usnea through a fine-mesh sieve lined with cheesecloth. Try to squeeze out as much of the tincture as you can.

Making a cup of usnea tea is unique as well. Ground 1 teaspoon of the herb, and pour just enough alcohol over it to saturate it. It's really not much, and the herb shouldn't be sitting in a puddle. Let it sit like this, covered, for 30 minutes. Then pour 6 ounces of boiling water over the herb and let steep for 15 minutes. This should cook off a good portion of the alcohol.

It may sound a little complicated, but it's really just a small bit of effort more for an effective antibiotic that is available almost everywhere in the United States.

Usnea can also absorb toxins from the environment. Play it safe, and only harvest lichens from at least 300 feet away from the side of a road, factory, or other source of waste.

Contraindications: Not for use during pregnancy. If possible, test on a small section of skin first, as usnea may cause contact dermatitis. Better to learn that now, with just a tiny section of redness, rather than applying it liberally to a wound and learning only then that you have an allergic skin reaction to it.

❦ VALERIAN
Valeriana officinalis

Parts Used: Root.

Actions: Analgesic, antispasmodic, anxiolytic, nervine, sedative.

Preparations: Fresh tincture (1:2 in 95% alcohol); dried tincture (1:5 in 75% alcohol); decoction.

Dose: 30 to 60 drops of tincture, 3 or 4 times daily; decoction, 2 or 3 times daily.

Uses: Valerian is the sleepy herb. It helps ease nerves and anxiety, induces sleepiness, and encourages the muscles to relax. At least, valerian does this for 90% of people. In 10% of the population, valerian acts like a stimulant.

The tincture dose suggested above is really just a standard guideline. Always start out with the least amount of valerian (or any herb for that matter). If you get no results, next time increase the dose by 5 drops. Continue this until you find your ideal dose, but don't exceed 60 drops.

Valerian is helpful with back pain and nerve pain. I suggest you use valerian when your day is essentially done and you can rest. Use a topical treatment, like cayenne, to address nerve and muscle pain during the day.

Contraindications: This really depends upon how valerian affects you. If it causes drowsiness, do not operate vehicles or heavy equipment.

❧ WHITE WILLOW
Salix alba

Parts Used: Inner bark.

Actions: Analgesic, anti-inflammatory, antirheumatic, febrifuge.

Preparations: Fresh tincture (1:2 in 95% alcohol); dried tincture (1:5 in 50% alcohol); decoction.

Dose: 30 to 60 drops of tincture, 3 to 4 times daily; 2 to 4 cups of decoction daily.

Uses: White willow is sometimes thought of as "herbal aspirin." One of its constituents, salicin, is metabolized into salicylic acid in the human body. This acid has been synthesized into the active ingredient in aspirin, acetylsalicylic acid.

However, there are some major differences between aspirin and white willow. The amount of salicin in white willow is far lower than the amount of acetylsalicylic acid in aspirin. In reality, there is very little salicin in white willow.

This may mean that another constituent within the inner bark of white willow is responsible for the bark's pain-relieving properties. It may also mean the synergistic nature of all the constituents is required to produce pain relief.

Yet the effect of white willow bark in relieving pain is quite similar to that of aspirin. Everybody reacts differently, but if I had to make any generalities about my experiences, I would say that white willow begins to relieve pain in about the same time as aspirin, although it takes a little longer for the pain relief to reach its peak. However, the overall effect of white willow seems to last longer than aspirin.

In studies involving white willow, there was a very low instance of allergic reactions or stomach discomfort (very common with aspirin). White willow also lacked the blood-thinning action found in aspirin.

While there has been research demonstrating white willow's effectiveness as a pain reliever, and showing differences between white willow and aspirin, there have not been enough studies to say that white willow won't carry some of the same risks as aspirin. So even though the amount of acetylsalicylic acid in aspirin is many times more than is found in white willow, and even though white willow bark has not demonstrated the same blood-thinning properties, those factors are not enough to base certain safety decisions on.

For example, aspirin is contraindicated in children with a fever or infection because it may lead to Reye's syndrome. Although white willow contains a small amount of salicin, a different chemical than acetylsalicylic acid, giving white willow bark tincture or tea to a child with an active infection is not recommended. For pain relief without an active infection, white willow bark is a safe remedy for children. Be sure to look for signs of infection, including:

+ fever

+ red streaks extending from an injured area

+ increasing pain, redness, swelling, or warmth around effected area

+ pus draining from an effected area

For adults with no aspirin allergy, white willow provides an effective, lasting pain reliever that is easier on the stomach than aspirin. White willow is safe for long-term use.

Contraindications: Not for people who are allergic to aspirin. Not for use during pregnancy. Not for use during breastfeeding. Not for use in children with a fever (which may indicate an infection).

YARROW
Achillea millefolium

Parts Used: Flowers, leaves.

Actions: Antiperspirant, astringent, diaphoretic, styptic, tonic, vulnerary.

Preparations: Fresh tincture from flowers (1:2 in 95% alcohol); dried tincture from flowers (1:5 in 75% alcohol); tisane from flowers; poultice from leaves.

Dose: 30 to 60 drops of tincture, 3 to 6 times daily, frequency depending on the purpose; 2 to 3 cups of tisane daily.

Uses: Yarrow is a complex herb made up of many active constituents. Yet yarrow has two primary Uses: to stop bleeding and to sweat out a fever.

The tincture can be applied topically, or the flowers can be made into a poultice, to stop a wound from bleeding. The tincture taken internally can help get internal bleeding under control. Yarrow also helps slow down an overly heavy menstrual cycle.

Yarrow is sometimes used by midwives in case of hemorrhage during or after birth. Another herb used in this manner is shepherd's purse (Capsella bursa-pastoris).

Having the ability to stop internal bleeding, or stop the bleeding of a deep wound, is lifesaving. I always carry yarrow in my herbal kit.

The tea has a different function. A tisane of yarrow flowers induces a sweat and effectively sweats out a fever.

Contraindications: Not for use with children. Not for use during pregnancy (except during labor and postpartum emergencies). Do not use while breastfeeding.

CHAPTER 5

HERBAL FIRST AID KIT

Most disasters—such as a hurricane, an earthquake, or limited civil unrest over a local tragedy—are short-term. But for the purposes of this book, I am assuming the worst-case scenario; namely, a long-term crisis with no hospitals, no pharmacies, and no trained medical professionals. You are the help you will need.

In a worst-case disaster, wounds will be a fact of life. People will be bitten, bruised, burned, blistered, and bleeding far more often than occurs today. And if you haven't had enough alliteration yet, there will be more pokes, prods, and punctures than ever before.

We will be outside more, moving more, lifting more, walking on uneven ground more, hunting more, and farming more. We will spend more time with biting insects and animals. We will be using more wood to heat our homes. We'll be doing a whole lot more cooking, and doing it most likely with wood, although there are good solar options as well.

There will be disagreements leading more readily to physical altercations. There will be people who did not prepare and are desperate and will try to take what you have set aside for yourself and your loved ones. Finally, there will be dishonorable folks whose plan it was all along to take what others have.

Civil unrest is to be expected in a worst-case scenario, with violence erupting suddenly and with frequency. Although there are many good books, classes, videos, and other instructional materials to help you prep for those scenarios, this discussion will focus on what happens after the dust settles, specifically acute care and recovery from injuries.

I strongly recommend taking a wilderness first aid course, which typically goes further than a standard first aid course. I maintain current information on both free and fee-based medical preparedness training, with and without herbs, on my website (www.HerbalPrepper.com) that is worth checking regularly.

In this book, my job is to provide you with herbal alternatives that you can grow and craft on your own without outside suppliers or supplies.

ADMINISTERING FIRST AID

Often, first aid instruction makes the assumption that you know what happened or that the person affected can tell you what happened. That may not always be the case. For example, if you happen to come home and find that the wood stove has burned out, the house is cold, and your partner is on the floor unconscious, you have a mystery to solve before you can help. If you come across someone who has collapsed in the snow, there's a shovel nearby, and the person seems to be dressed warmly enough, you have another mystery to solve.

Always make sure that you are safe before attempting to help. Check for animals, people, electrical wires, traps, and anything else that stands out as a potential hazard. You will do no one any good if you are also injured. You will also make the job of anyone coming to your aid harder now that there are two injured people.

Look for signs of what happened. Is the person bleeding? Is he or she breathing, and is there a pulse? Does it look like a fall? Do you smell alcohol? Ask if the person can hear you.

In the case of the person lying unconscious on the floor, there are many possibilities. He or she could have been knocked out by an intruder or overcome by carbon monoxide. Or, the person could have been bitten by a spider that had crept close to the stove seeking heat.

The person collapsed in the snow could have fallen victim to hypothermia or might have had a heart attack while shoveling.

You may not know exactly what is going on in every situation. But if you have solid first aid skills, know how to do chest compressions, understand how to clear a spine, know how to stop bleeding by applying pressure, and have an array of herbal medicines to pick from, you'll be better equipped to handle more health emergencies than most people in a worst-case scenario.

A FEW WORDS ABOUT YOUR FIRST AID KIT

Containers. I love my beautiful glass jars and bottles. However, they have no business in an emergency kit that will be banged around, bumped, tossed, and who knows what else. I keep most of the liquids in my kit in HDPE plastic. The material was designed for caustic liquids. For milder liquids, I do use some other types of plastic. For the short-term emergency use for which these formulas are intended, I'm not worried about anything leaching.

Herbs. The formulas included here are made from dried herbs. I made this decision so that even if you are reading this book in November, or if you live in a small apartment in the middle of the city, you can still order the herbs and make these remedies. If you are fortunate enough to have access to fresh plant material, just use the information from other chapters to make your adjustments.

Of course, if you use the simpler's method (page 32), or if you stick to 80 or 100 proof vodka, then you can ignore some of the specifics in the formulas. Your creations will be more intuitive than measured, and that's perfectly fine. You will still end up with effective remedies.

The formulas call for some herbs that are not included in Chapter 4, Materia Medica. There are many more herbs than the 50 that I included, but I may never have finished this book without setting a limit. There will be information on my website about other herbs. Perhaps, someday, there will be time to write an inclusive herbal tome.

Labeling. Yes, I do repeat myself about labeling each bottled remedy. I promise you, in a couple of months you will not remember what is in that bottle. I've been there. Every herbalist has. And if you don't know what it is, you can't use it. So I'm hoping my repetitiveness prevents problems for you.

DOSAGE CONSIDERATIONS

Some family members may need different doses than the standard ones I've listed. Let's look at dosing considerations for "special populations" such as children, pregnant and nursing women, overweight adults, and the elderly.

Children. Several methods of calculating a child's dosage have evolved over the years. Three of the most common are Cowling's rule, Clark's rule, and Young's rule.

RULE	EQUATION
Cowling's	Child's age at next birthday ÷ 24 = child's dosage *Example dosage for a 3-year-old going to be 4 at next birthday:* 4 ÷ 24 = approximately ⅙ of adult dosage
Clark's	Child's weight ÷ 150 = child's dosage *Example dosage for a 75-pound child:* 75 ÷ 150 = ½ of adult dosage
Young's	Child's age ÷ (child's age + 12) = child's dosage *Example dosage for a 6-year-old:* 6 ÷ (6+12) or 6 ÷ 18 = ⅓ of adult dosage

Pregnant and Nursing Women. There are no unique dosing considerations for pregnant or nursing women. However, many herbs are not appropriate during pregnancy, and some herbs are appropriate only at certain times during pregnancy. For instance, black cohosh is not appropriate for muscle soreness during pregnancy. But to help start and establish labor, black cohosh is appropriate. Herbs that shouldn't be used during pregnancy are covered in Chapter 4, Materia Medica. Be sure to check contraindications before including herbs in remedies for pregnant or nursing women.

Overweight Adults. It has been my experience that larger adults, whether by height or weight, do need stronger or more frequent doses. But you have to be careful since an overweight person doesn't necessarily have larger internal organs. You can't just double the dosage from a 150-pound person to a 300-pound person. Be mindful of other health issues, especially related to blood pressure, blood glucose, and hormonal balance.

I've found it better to add an extra dose at the same strength, observe the results, and adjust as needed.

The Elderly. Dosage considerations for the elderly are highly individualized. Some people remain active, are connected to their communities, participate in civic and charitable events, continue to drive, have good eyesight, and show few to no signs of chronic illness. They don't require anything different from any other healthy adult.

Unfortunately, this is not the norm for the elderly population in the United States. Advanced age and illness have almost become synonymous. If you are dealing with someone who is frail, focus on nourishing and tonic herbs. Many elderly are cold all the time because of poor circulation. Chronic illness is common, so be aware of arthritis and diabetes. Also keep in mind that cell regeneration slows down with age, and wound healing may take a long time. The skin becomes thinner as it ages, is more easily broken, and may take longer to heal. You may want to consider topicals, such as lotions, creams, and salves, in which you incorporate the pain-relieving herbs.

Just remember that 100% natural lotions and creams contain water. Without a preservative, they will grow mold, bacteria, and all sorts of funky things. Some essential oils, depending upon which ones, may preserve a lotion for up to a month, but that same strength of oils may also be too intense for an elderly person. Keep lotions in a cool, dark place, and make them in small batches so they are used up before they grow something unpleasant.

Following are some common injuries and ailments you may encounter, as well as suggestions for what to keep in your first aid kit to treat them.

❦ ALLERGY AND ANAPHYLAXIS ❦ (SEVERE)

Anaphylaxis is a severe allergic reaction, often to foods like shellfish or nuts, or in some cases to bee or wasp stings. If you know you have a severe allergy, especially if you have to carry an EpiPen, you absolutely have to have a plan B.

One suggestion for prevention is to eat a diet high in omega 3 fatty acids. Some studies show that animals on a high omega 3 diet had a better survival rate after anaphylaxis than those who ate more omega 6 fatty acids. I wouldn't count on that exclusively, but eating plenty of omega 3 fatty acids won't hurt. Plus there are many benefits in consuming omega 3 fatty acids, including lowering inflammation, helping relieve stiff arthritic joints, and lowering elevated triglycerides.

Ma Huang (Ephedra)

Normally, anaphylaxis is treated with an EpiPen, which delivers epinephrine to stop the reaction. Ephedrine is similar to epinephrine, and ma huang (Ephedra sinica) contains ephedrine.[11]

See page 122 for dosing instructions and precautions. Do be aware that ephedra can raise blood pressure.

Lobelia Tincture

Another option is lobelia tincture, which is beneficial for asthma. It is also a help in at least certain cases of anaphylaxis. A dose equivalent to 10 to 40 drops of lobelia extract should be administered every hour up to 6 hours, depending on the individual's needs.[12] Given its effectiveness for asthma, I suspect it would be useful for other types of anaphylaxis.

Food Allergy Herbal Formula

Finally, I present an option for you to investigate further. It has very promising research behind it, but the remedy is based in traditional Chinese medicine and I am not well versed in TCM. This formula has been shown to prevent anaphylaxis when people who are allergic to peanuts consume peanuts. It is based on the wu mei wan blend with two herbs (zhi fu zi and xi xin) left out of the formula, plus an herb called ling zhi added to the formula. Wu mei wan can be purchased as capsules

---

11   According to *The Merck Manual:* "Ephedrine has alpha and beta effects similar to epinephrine but differs from it in being effective orally, having a slower onset and longer duration of action, and a greater stimulant effect on the CNS, producing alertness, anxiety, insomnia, and tremor." Robert Porter, *The Merck Manual* (Whitehouse Station, NJ: Merck, 2011).

12   Finley Ellingwood, *The American Materia Medica, Therapeutics and Pharmacognosy* (Chicago: Ellingwood's Therapeutists, 1915).

online, as can ling zhi. The new formula is called FAHF-2 (FAHF stands for "Food Allergy Herbal Formula"). These are the percentages of the herbs used in FAHF-2:[13]

Ling zhi *(Ganoderma lucidum)*, 28.17%

Wu mei *(fructus pruni mume)*, 28.17%

Huang lian *(rhizoma coptidis)*, 8.46%

Ren shen *(radix ginseng)*, 8.45%

Huang bai *(cortex phellodendri)*, 5.63%

Gan jiang *(rhizoma zingiberis officinalis)*, 8.45%

Dang gui *(radix angelicae sinensis)*, 8.45%

Gui zhi *(ramulus cinnamomi cassiae)*, 2.81%

Chuan jiao *(pericarpium zanthoxyli bungeanum)*, 1.41%

I doubt that these herbs will be available for harvest here in the United States for use in a post-disaster scenario. However, you can purchase and stockpile them now, unlike an EpiPen and the follow-up antihistamine treatment.

The follow-up for any of these severe allergy options should be nettle and liver support. The liver manufactures antihistamine, and nettle provides antihistamine.

☙ ANTI-INFECTION SALVE ☙

This is perfect for all minor wounds, scrapes, small cuts, and other minor injuries. Any open wound can become infected. We tend not to worry about them in our sanitized, modern lives, but during a crisis even a small cut can turn deadly. If you see a red line tracing up from the wound, it's

---

13   This breakdown and further information on FAHF-2 can be found in the online magazine *Acupuncture Today*. Jake Paul Fratkin, "Stunning Herbal Formula Wins Recognition in the Western Medical Community," *Acupuncture Today* 6, no. 12 (2005). http://www.acupuncturetoday.com/archives2005/dec/12fratkin.html.

too late to use this salve as a preventive remedy. In this case, begin a course of sida tincture to prevent infection from spreading.

The amounts are variable, depending on how much you want to make at one time.

Olive oil	**Lavender flowers**	**Plantain leaves**
Thyme leaves	**Calendula flowers**	**Beeswax**

1 Infuse thyme, lavender, calendula, and plantain into olive oil. You can use any portions you wish, although I tend to do equal portions (example, ½ cup of each herb and cover in oil). You can do this individually or all at once. Infuse the herbs in oil either by maceration or in the slow cooker. If macerating, soak for 6 weeks. If using a slow cooker, set on low for 2 to 4 hours on warm (if your slow cooker has a warm setting) for up to 2 weeks.

2 Strain the herbs, and bottle the oil.

3 Using a double boiler, warm 8 fluid ounces of the infused oil and 2 tablespoons of beeswax until the wax has fully melted into the oil. Use low heat. Do not try to speed the melting by turning up the heat. You do not want to cook the oil.

4 Take the double boiler off the heat, and pour the liquid into jars or tins.

5 Allow to cool, and label the containers.

6 Add one container to your kit, and store the rest.

❦ ANTI-INFLAMMATORY CAPSULES ❦

This remedy requires a capsule machine, capsules, and powdered herbs. Although you may have to put in a little more labor to powder the herbs and fill the capsule machine with capsules, this is a highly convenient way to administer herbs.

4 parts ginger	**4 parts turmeric**	**1 part black pepper**

1 Follow the directions on your capsule machine.

Personal preference: I like to take two size 00 capsules (approximately 700 mg each) 3 to 6 times throughout the day to relieve inflammation.

INDIVIDUAL INFUSIONS V. COMBINED INFUSIONS

When you set up your home apothecary, you have a choice to make singles (individual extractions, like arnica infused oil or dandelion tincture) or blends (multiple herb extractions, like black cohosh, cramp bark, and white willow infused in oil together for an anti-inflammatory and antispasmodic massage oil or salve). Making singles gives you the widest range of options for use, while making blends saves a step toward making a final product. I personally prefer to make singles and blend the singles as needed, though I do set up a few blends of remedies I use a lot. This is a matter of personal preference, and there is no right or wrong way.

🐛 ANTI-PARASITIC/PROTOZOAN 🐛 TINCTURE

Access to clean water is vital. Lack of potable water can lead to a parasitic infection such as giardia or cryptosporidiosis. If you suspect this type of infection, try the following tincture blend.

1 part wormwood (*Artemisia absinthium*) tincture

1 part black walnut tincture (the green hulls)

1 part garlic tincture

1 part horseradish tincture

1 part milk thistle tincture

1 part cloves tincture

1 part thyme tincture

1 part berberine tincture (type local to you)

1 part ginger tincture

1   Blend these tinctures together.

2   Bottle, label, and add to your kit.

3   Take a standard 30 to 60 drop dose, 3 to 6 times per day, when symptoms of parasitic infection are present.

❦ ANTI-SCAR SALVE ❦

If a severe burn victim is lucky enough to survive the extensive trauma, there may be scarring. This salve may be able to help.

1 part rose hip seed oil (can substitute pumpkin seed oil if you don't have rose hip seed oil)

1 part St. John's wort infused oil

1 part comfrey infused oil

1 part plantain infused oil

1 tablespoon lanolin (if allergic, leave out)

1 tablespoon beeswax

3 tablespoons honey

30 to 60 drops lavender essential oil

1 Either purchase or press rose hip seed oil. This is a wonderful skin-healing oil.

2 Make infused oils of St. John's wort, comfrey, and plantain, either individually or all together. I suggest individually.

3 Blend equal parts of these oils and the rose hip seed oil.

4 Melt the beeswax and lanolin into 1 cup of the blended oil slowly on low heat to avoid cooking the oil.

5 When the wax and lanolin are completely melted, remove from the heat.

6 Once the wax has begun to cool, add the honey. This may take some stirring to fully incorporate, or use an immersion blender.

7 Add lavender essential oil, and incorporate into the salve.

8 Scoop into containers, and label. Put one container in your kit, and store the rest.

9 Massage often to soften scar tissue.

❦ ANTIBACTERIAL TINCTURE ❦

Ideally, I prefer to know more about an infection before selecting an herbal remedy. That may not always be possible, especially in an emergency without the benefit of diagnostics. To take this one step further, even if I know exactly what the infection is once I arrive on scene, I can't carry dozens of tincture bottles in my kit. My solution is an "everything but the kitchen sink" approach. I make each tincture individually and then blend them together for use in the kit.

It is important to note that the terms "antibacterial" and "antiviral" do not mean "kills all bacteria" or "kills all viruses." They are effective against certain bacteria or viruses. The ideal would be to know specifically which bacteria or virus this or that herb has been shown effective against, and to be at home with all of your herbal tinctures at your disposal. However, in an emergency, and for simplicity's sake, the easiest approach is to have a single antibacterial formula that is effective against a very wide range of bacteria, and the same goes for having a single antiviral formula (follow the antibacterial formula below). This way, you can address more infections while carrying fewer bottles.

4 parts sida tincture, aerial parts

4 parts sweet annie tincture *(Artemisia annua)*

3 parts *Echinacea angustifolia* root tincture

2 parts juniper berry tincture

2 parts usnea tincture

2 parts garlic clove tincture

1 part black pepper tincture

1 Blend these tinctures together.

2 Bottle, label, and add to your kit.

3 Administer a standard 30 to 60 drop dose, 3 to 6 times per day, when symptoms of bacterial infection are present.

❦ ANTIVIRAL TINCTURE ❦

Taking the same approach for an antiviral tincture as I do with Antibacterial Tincture, this is the formula I carry.

3 parts Chinese skullcap tincture

3 parts red sage *(Salvia miltiorrhiza)* tincture

3 parts dong quai *(Angelica sinensis)* tincture

2 parts elderberry tincture

2 parts echinacea tincture

1 part ginger tincture

1 part licorice tincture

1 Blend these tinctures together.

2 Bottle, label, and add to your kit.

3 Administer a standard 30 to 60 drop dose, 3 to 6 times per day, when symptoms of viral infection are present.

❧ BURN CARE ❧

Burns are classified by degrees that correlate to layers of the skin. First-degree burns affect the epidermis, second-degree burns impact the dermis, and third-degree burns reach to the subcutaneous, also called the hypodermis. There is also a fourth degree, a full-thickness burn through the skin layers down to muscle and/or bone.

First-degree burns are often sunburns. Trust me when I tell you that I'm as white as a ghost, and sunburns are serious, painful burns that sometimes progress into second-degree burns. I've had a lot of experience with burns, where people have been seriously hurt or scarred. I've been the first responder in a remote area and seen hands and limbs that had been burned in a campfire. Every type of burn is serious business.

Burns can be caused by heat, chemicals, electricity, or radiation. Heat might be fire, or it could be a steaming pot of water that gets knocked off the stove (always turn your pot handles inward when cooking). Chemical burns require thorough flushing, and when you think you have flushed enough, go ahead and do it again. If you do not remove all of the chemical, a first-degree chemical burn can turn into a fourth-degree one.

With electrical burns, be very, very careful to ensure that you do not get electrocuted yourself. Use a wooden broom handle to move a wire if necessary, and do not step into water around downed or connected wires. Be aware of your surroundings, especially if there is bad weather. The last type of burn is a radiation burn. Although radiation burns could be from medical treatments, they are almost always sunburns.

The first order of business is to stop the extent of the damage. This might consist of smothering the person with a blanket to put out flames. At some point and very quickly, you need to cool down the tissues. This is most often done by running cool, not cold, water over the burn. Remove any clothing or jewelry that might hold heat. Anything that covers the burn site will retain heat. Do not apply oil or butter to the burn. It will only hold in heat and cause the burn to progress. The only exception is if the burn is from tar, because no amount of water will get tar off. Go ahead and use the fat to remove the tar, and then immediately begin cooling the skin with water.

There are many ways to determine the depth of a burn. But in an emergency, the easiest thing to remember is that pain is actually good. It means that the burn has not gone beyond second degree and the roots of the nerves are still intact. If the person has no pain, the burn is third or fourth degree.

You will need to assess a burn victim for the extent of the depth (degree) of the burn, as well as the percentage of body burned. Normally, the "rule of nines" is used to assess the percentage of body burned. This is a method used by paramedics where limbs, the torso, and head are assigned percentages based on the number nine. But unless you do this often, it's easy to forget what limb equals what percentage during an actual emergency. A simpler approach is to remember that the palm of your hand is approximately 1% of the body. You can use that as a guide in determining the percentage burned. If more than 10% of the body is burned, you can expect difficulty in regulating body temperature, keeping the person hydrated, and preventing infection. Be on the lookout for shock and sudden drops in blood pressure from fluids leaving the vascular spaces.

Second-degree burns may blister. If this happens, leave them alone unless they are cutting off circulation. Intact blisters act as a sterile bandage. Eventually, the fluid inside will get reabsorbed. If a blister pops, then you need to debride it (remove the damaged tissue). Clean it with Wound Wash (page 161), and be sure to get out the thick fluid. Using a scalpel, cut the dead skin layer as close to the new skin layer as possible to prevent it from getting caught or pulling. Cutting it off as close to the healthy skin as possible without cutting into that healthy skin allows for new skin growth. Treat this area as you would any other open wound.

The only other time debriding comes into play is when there is an eschar, or dead tissue. It must come off. If it is a large area, debriding can be done in stages. But if you do not remove the dead tissue, it can breed infection, including gangrene, and the body can develop sepsis.

You already have everything you need in your kit to treat the burn. Clean any wound with Wound Wash. You can also use it to spray a sunburn for relief. With any open wound from a blister, you can use Anti-Scar Salve (page 128), Wound Powder: Antibacterial (page 161), or Antibacterial Tincture (page 128). For any full-thickness burn, apply raw honey or Wound, Burn, or "SHTF" Honey (page 159), and cover with a bandage. For all burns, change the bandage daily to see how the burn is healing and to check for infection.

Caring for full-thickness burns can take months. There is a lot more to caring for a full-thickness burn victim than there is to providing first aid. Some of the most important points to remember are:

+ Be alert for unsafe drops in blood pressure from dehydration. Without the skin as a barrier, moisture evaporates from the body. Keep the person covered, and monitor his or her blood pressure.

+ Encourage drinking fluids with rehydration salts.

If this is insufficient to keep the person hydrated, and you do not know how to start an IV, then you may want to rig up a drip of normal saline (it's the easiest saline to make at home and can be preserved in mason jars by pressure canning) to get into the burn victim with an enema. This method, which provides fluids rectally, was done prior to development of IV fluids through a line.

In addition to herbs to help tissue repair, a burn victim requires a lot of food energy to repair tissue: 5,000 calories per day of nutrient-dense foods.

🦌 COLD WEATHER INJURY CARE 🦌

Cold weather injuries include the following:

+ Injuries to the extremities.

+ Injuries to the core.

+ Infections from dead tissue.

Cold weather injuries usually bring to mind such conditions as frostbite, hypothermia, chilblains, and trench foot. Frostbite, chilblains, and trench foot are injuries to the extremities. Hypothermia is an injury to the core.

Prevention is key. Keep warm by wearing layers. Wool is an excellent choice because it stays warm even when wet. Keep extra wool socks in the bugout bag.

If you find someone unconscious in the snow, do not rub that person vigorously. You could actually cause a heart attack. Don't rub the extremities, for example, fingers and the tips of ears, either. If frozen, they could break right off!

One thing I want to stress: Never give cayenne or ginger to someone who has been out in the cold until you know their core is warm. If you start applying cayenne salve to the extremities, or giving cayenne or ginger internally to help "get the blood pumping," then you are taking body heat away from the core. Give cayenne or ginger only when you know the core is warm.

The best thing you can do is to get the person warm. If you have only a blanket, then put that blanket between the individual and the ground, and use your body heat to help warm the person. At some point, however, you will have to get the person to shelter.

Children (okay, and some adults too) just don't know that they are too cold to be safe outside because they are having so much fun in the snow. If they begin to shiver, that's a sign that their body temperature is dropping, and they need to get warm right away. When the shivering stops, it is not because they have adjusted to the outside temperature. It is just the next step in hypothermia.

For hypothermia, you must warm the body. Sitting by a heater, sipping a hot beverage, like broth or herbal tea, can help warm up the core. Provide blankets, body heat, or even a lukewarm bath at 105°F. Hypothermia is a dangerous situation and can progress into serious medical conditions, such as cardiac arrest, kidney problems, and pancreatitis. Without access to medical care, do take every precaution to avoid hypothermia.

You can treat damage or wounds to the extremities exactly as you do a burn. If there is a wound, wash it. If there is a blister (chilblains, most likely), leave it alone unless it bursts or cuts off circulation. If there is frostbite, stop the damage from spreading and warm up the body. Just don't rub the body to warm it.

If there is dead tissue, it must be debrided. Otherwise, it could become gangrenous, and septicemia or sepsis will follow.

❦ CONSTIPATION ❦

Having the problem opposite to diarrhea can be just as serious. Constipation can be brought on by stress, change in diet, and lack of fluids. These conditions can easily happen simultaneously during a crisis.

This is one of many reasons why we should eat what we store and store what we eat. Yes, you can have a large stockpile of freeze-dried foods as a backup. But it is far better in the long run to dehydrate, ferment, and freeze (if possible) your own food storage and eat from it regularly. You can ensure there is plenty of fiber and moisture, which are often lacking in prepackaged meals.

If dehydration is the issue, increase fluids. If being sedentary, perhaps due to injury, is the issue, find a way to move without aggravating the injury. An enema may be necessary if the person is impacted. However, with plenty of fluids, movement, and a few natural helpers, most of the time an enema shouldn't be necessary.

Natural remedies that can help relieve constipation include:

+ Yellow Dock and Molasses Syrup (page 193)
+ Traditional Fire Cider (page 167)
+ Fruit juices
+ Fermented foods or probiotic supplement
+ Marshmallow root cold infusion

Senna is an herbal option for constipation relief, but it is a laxative, unlike the more gentle options above. I find it far too harsh and had intense cramping whenever I tried it. Senna has a role to play, but I don't use it unless truly necessary.

❦ DENTAL INFECTION TINCTURE ❦ AND MOUTHWASH

Few things can stop a person in his or her tracks like an oral infection. A simple tincture made with some of the ingredients for the Herbal Throat Spray used directly at the site of pain or infection in the mouth can go a long way toward relieving the pain and resolving the infection. You can also use it as a mouthwash, if you find yourself without toothpaste, or if your gums or the inside of the mouth are injured.

If doctors are hard to come by in a worst-case survival situation, you can bet that dentists will also be scarce. If you have any option for getting antibiotics or having a dentist look at your tooth, do so. This tincture is appropriate for any type of mouth pain, and it can be used directly on a dental abscess. An infection from a dental abscess can migrate to the heart, where it can be fatal.

2 fluid ounces spilanthes tincture

2 fluid ounces echinacea tincture

2 fluid ounces berberine tincture (type local to you)

2 fluid ounces clove tincture

1 Mix the tinctures together.

2 For infections, such as an abscess, apply as needed directly to the abscess. The abscess may need to be drained and an herbal antibiotic, like Antibacterial Tincture (see page 128), may be necessary until you are able to get to a dentist.

3 Fill a spray bottle, label it, and add it to your kit. Keep the rest in storage.

To make a mouthwash, add 8 ounces of clean water. The alcohol in the tinctures should be sufficient to preserve the wash. Spilanthes induces saliva production, so you shouldn't need more water than that. Swish around the mouth and spit.

❦ DIARRHEA, DEHYDRATION, AND ❦ DIY ORAL REHYDRATION SALTS

Diarrhea can be caused by parasites, bacteria, or viruses. As well as being extremely uncomfortable, diarrhea can be dangerous because of the massive loss of fluids and nutrients. Most people recover providing they remain hydrated.

In addition to the parasitic infections giardia and cryptosporidiosis, two of the most common viral infections causing diarrhea are norovirus and rotavirus.

Rotavirus is still a big killer of children worldwide in third world conditions. Keep in mind that if economic collapse or any of the potential disasters that preppers keep a close watch on were to happen, those same conditions may become common here in the United States. The source for viral infection is usually contaminated waste, which clings to plants. The incubation period is 2 days, followed by vomiting, then 4 to 8 days of watery diarrhea, low fever, and possible dehydration.

Norovirus is responsible for 90% of all non-bacterial gastroenteritis worldwide and 50% of all infection in the United States. Sources of norovirus are contaminated water, person-to-person transmission, and food handled by an infected person, which is common in closed populations such as nursing homes, cruise ships, prisons, and schools. Norovirus is highly infectious. The symptoms and incubation period are the same as for rotavirus. One difference is that norovirus is still contagious for 2 weeks after symptoms have abated, while the rotavirus is only contagious for 2 to 10 days of onset of symptoms. In a post-disaster scenario we wouldn't have access to a lab to determine whether the outbreak was norovirus or rotavirus, so it is safer to act as if all infections are norovirus and to assume victims are infectious for 2 weeks after their symptoms subside.

In general, tannin-containing herbs, fruits, and bark inactivate viral gastroenteritis diseases. Tannin sources include cranberry, blackberry root, pomegranate, oak bark, and pine needles. Cranberry, which is easy to store, can be used as juice, but it must be unsweetened. You might be able to get away with cranberry sweetened with grape juice, but absolutely no added sugars. That would make the diarrhea worse.

Other herbs that can help include licorice, especially for rotavirus, and *Potentilla erecta* and *P. tormentil,* which boast 18% to 30% tannins.[14]

Salmonella

Salmonella is a common infection that packs a wallop and now shows some drug resistance. It is found all over grocery store shelves and in all conventionally raised chicken and eggs. Salmonella is in contaminated food packaging plants, which is how it ends up in raw foods like sprouts and spinach. If ever there was an argument for keeping your own chickens, salmonella is it.

Here are a few "fun facts" about salmonella:

+ It can live outside a host for years.

+ Freezing does not kill it.

+ Heating does kill it (either 130°F for 1 hour or 170°F for 10 minutes).

+ Salmonella symptoms include diarrhea, vomiting, severe abdominal cramps, and, in severe cases, sepsis and infection of other organs. Herbs and natural remedies that are helpful include:

  + Juniper berries and needles

  + Berberine herb

  + Sida tincture

---

14 In Mrs. Grieve's book, *A Modern Herbal,* she provides a remedy for dysentery as follows from "Compound Powder of Tormentil:" "A very reliable medicine in diarrhea and dysentery. Powdered Tormentil, 1 OZ; Powdered Galangal, 1 OZ.; Powdered Marshmallow root, 1 OZ.; Powdered Ginger, 4 drachms. An infusion is made of the powdered ingredients by pouring 1 pint of boiling water upon them, allowing to cool and then straining the liquid. Dose, 1 or 2 fluid drachms, every 15 minutes, till the pain is relieved—then take three or four times a day." Margaret Grieve, *A Modern Herbal* (New York: Dover Publications, 1971).

- + Activated charcoal
- + Rhodiola, licorice, and ginger juice (or ginger tincture instead of the juice)

E. Coli

E. coli is another common intestinal infection. It comes from the same sorts of places as salmonella. E. coli has several strains, but if you are without a lab, you won't know which strain you have. Symptoms include hemorrhagic diarrhea, severe intestinal cramps, and even kidney failure. I would approach a suspected E. coli event the same way as I would salmonella, but I would add oak bark decoction for the tannins, echinacea tincture, a tincture of ginger, licorice, and reishi, and nettle seed tincture.

Oral Rehydration Salts

In any case of diarrhea, you may have to make a batch of oral rehydration salts (ORS). You can use any clean water plus regular white sugar and table salt. You can substitute honey for the sugar, Celtic sea salt for table salt, and coconut water for tap water. Here are two recipes that I like.

2 tablespoons sugar + ½ teaspoon sea salt + 1 quart water

OR

½ teaspoon sea salt + 2 tablespoons honey + tiny bit of warm coconut water to help warm and thin the honey, making it easier to mix + 1 quart of coconut water

Give ORS in 1-cup doses after each episode of diarrhea.

❦ EAR INFECTION DROPS ❦

Ear infections tend to be a childhood problem, but not always. Some adults still get ear infections. I used to get them well into my mid-twenties. If you are bugging out with children, however, ear infections can be a real problem.

Some of the classic herbal remedies include garlic infused oil and mullein flower infused oil. You can use them individually or combine them.

However, I am not a big fan of garlic infused oil unless it has just been made in a slow cooker on low for 4 hours and allowed to cool. Garlic infused oil has a tendency toward botulism, and there is a small chance of botulism through topical application. It is very slight, and is usually more apt to happen in massive injuries where crushing is involved. I just don't feel comfortable with the risk when it comes to kids, especially when other remedies are available.

Mullein flower infused oil is my preferred choice for ear drops. I have also heard of other herbalists using echinacea and bee balm *(Monarda)* in their ear drops.

Mullein flowers   **Olive oil (enough to completely cover your mullein flowers)**

1   Infuse the mullein flowers in the olive oil.

2   Strain out the flowers, reserving the infused oil.

3   Bottle and label the oil.

4   Store the bulk of the oil, and bottle a very small amount for your kit. Oil is used only a few drops at a time.

5   To use, gently warm the oil by holding the bottle in warm water. Use either an orifice reducer (the type used in essential oil bottling) or a small HDPE bottle and a disposable plastic pipette. At home, it's far easier to use a glass pipette without risk of breaking it.

6   Drop 3 or 4 drops of oil onto the side of the ear canal, and allow the oil to make its own way down.

7   Apply 4 to 6 times per day until symptoms stop.

Do not use if the eardrum is perforated.

❦ EARACHE REMEDY ❦

My favorite earache remedy by far is lavender essential oil. I like it even more than the ear drops made from mullein flowers. For the kids, I take a cotton ball and work it into an earplug. Then I add a drop or two of lavender essential oil to the part of the plug that will stick into the ear but doesn't actually go far into the ear canal. The vapors from the lavender oil make their way to the infection, providing relief. This is even better if you can have the child rest the infected ear on a hot water bottle wrapped in towels for protection. Between the warmth and the lavender essential oil, this remedy should provide relief from both pain and infection without having to actually drop anything into the ear.

❦ EYE INFECTION ❦ WASH/COMPRESS

An eye infection is never pleasant. Conjunctivitis, probably the most common eye infection, is often called "pink eye" because of how red and irritated the eye becomes. It is highly contagious. In an environment where unclean hands touch the face, odds are high that you or someone in your group will develop an eye infection. Always remember to wash your hands as often as possible and avoid touching the face.

This blend of herbs can be made as an infusion, or you can make a decoction of your berberine herb, add the other herbs and allow them to steep, covered, for 15 minutes, and then strain out all the herbs, reserving the liquid. Apply with a towel used as a cooling compress. It can also be used with an eye cup to rinse foreign matter out of the eye. Be absolutely sure to strain all herbal material when making this wash. The last thing anyone needs is a tiny bit of plant material scratching the cornea. Be vigilant in straining with a fine-mesh sieve, a piece of nylon stocking, or a muslin bag.

1 part berberine (type local to you)	1 part calendula	2 parts eyebright *(Euphrasia)*
	1 part echinacea	

1   Make small batches because the wash will keep for only 2 to 3 days in the refrigerator.

2   Make a decoction of berberine.

3   Add the remaining herbs and steep, covered, for at least 30 minutes.

4   Strain out all plant matter, and store in the refrigerator.

5   Use as an eye wash, or mix with witch hazel and use as a compress.

For an emergency first aid kit, store the herbal blend in a jar and make a strong tea only when needed. Strain through a muslin bag, and use as either a wash or a compress.

❦ FRACTURE AND BROKEN ❦ BONES POULTICE

Typically, a broken bone is obvious. A fracture is less so. Both are serious, painful injuries. Some are far more complicated to deal with than others. Properly setting a bone is a specialized skill, and I strongly encourage you to take advanced first aid and emergency training before attempting it. There are dangers beyond having a bone heal improperly (and having to rebreak and reset it). Depending on where the break is, moving the person may cause massive bleeding (upper thigh), or may worsen the break and cause fractured shards to migrate.

It may not be immediately clear if there is fracturing. For example, it is very easy to fracture some of the small bones in your foot if you fall and severely sprain your ankle. In that case, the treatment for the sprain and the fracture are the same. Immobilize the ankle and foot with either a compression bandage or an air cast if you have one. Keep the foot elevated whenever possible, apply ice and an herbal poultice, and give an herbal pain reliever if needed. A similar treatment can be done for a hand or forearm by immobilizing a suspected fracture with an air cast.

Once the bone is safely and properly set, herbal treatment for bone healing can begin. This takes the form of poultices, nutritional support for the bones, and herbs to help relieve the pain. I would use the exact same poultice as for Sprains and Bruises Salve/Poultice (page 155). If the skin is broken, leave out the arnica and add more comfrey and goldenrod. I would also give the following nutritional syrup.

NUTRITIONAL SYRUP

2 parts nettle leaves	1 part burdock root	1 part red clover
2 parts horsetail	1 part rose hips	*(Trifolium pratense)*
(Equisetum arvense)		Molasses

1   Blend the herbs together.

2   Make a decoction of the herbs using 1 cup of water and ½ cup of the herbal blend. You should end up with approximately ½ cup of liquid or slightly less, depending on how well you drain the herbs.

3   Strain out the herbs, and combine with blackstrap molasses to reach a volume of 1 full cup.

4   Bottle, label, and store in the refrigerator. The syrup will keep for only a few days at room temperature. If it is summer or you live somewhere hot, try making a double decoction to reduce the water content, but it is still best stored in the refrigerator. If grabbing your kit, add this syrup to the kit just before leaving.

5   There will also be pain and inflammation to deal with. See the tinctures for major and minor pain on pages 147 and 148.

❦ HEART ATTACK CARE ❦

One thing I foresee happening a lot, unfortunately, is heart attack. People who are sedentary suddenly being required to move more just to survive, people with hypertension thrown into stressful situations, laboring outdoors in the cold, and a dozen other possibilities will make heart attacks even more common during a disaster than they are now.

I've read about and know several people who have used cayenne tincture during a heart attack. And while it's wonderful that they survived, there are issues with using cayenne, even if it potentially played a role in their survival. Cayenne is one of the fastest acting-vasodilating and blood-thinning herbs. It makes some sense to use during a heart attack for those reasons. But how do you know for sure whether the person had a heart attack in the first place?

Let's say you come upon someone who is unconscious. You call out, check for signs of life, check for spinal injury, support/stabilize the neck, and try to piece together what happened. The person may have had a heart attack, or may have tripped and fallen, hitting his or her head. Or the individual may have had a stroke or a ruptured aneurysm. Thinning the blood may be the exact opposite of what you want.

There are so many scenarios that could bring you in contact with an unconscious person. If you know the person, and you know of a history of heart attacks or some cardiovascular problem (especially if you just heard complaints of heart attack symptoms), and you see that individual fall to the ground, and you feel confident that a heart attack occurred, then it may make sense to give cayenne tincture.

I can't make this call for you, but I do suggest learning the signs of a heart attack as opposed to a brain hemorrhage, ruptured aneurysm, and so on. Of course, this only helps if the episode takes place right in front of you and you know the individual's health history. Personally, I would focus more on beginning chest compressions. Hopefully, someone will arrive or you will have on hand a portable defibrillator. Unfortunately, most people do not regain consciousness through chest compressions alone. Chest compressions are important to help keep a person going until a defibrillator or other intervention can be applied. Portable and home defibrillators are available for anyone to purchase. Amazon often runs sales on them. If you have heart disease in your family, it may be worth the expense.

Afterward, however, hawthorn berry tincture can be a great help in healing any damage to the heart suffered during a heart attack. Hawthorn berry tincture (page 86) is a great cardiac tonic for both preventive care and aftercare healing.

❦ INTERNAL BLEEDING TINCTURE ❦

This tincture may be of use when you see signs of internal bleeding, which will vary depending on where the bleed is. For example, bleeding from the kidney or bladder would result in blood in the urine. Intestinal and stomach bleeding would show blood in the stools. Bleeding in the liver or spleen causes abdominal pain and swelling. Other symptoms of internal bleeding include low blood pressure, dizziness when standing, and bleeding from any body orifice.

Yarrow is called "the battlefield herb" for a reason. It is known for its ability to control the blood—to stop bleeding as well as prevent dangerous clots. You can use yarrow picked straight out of the ground, the flower ground up as a wound powder, or in the following tincture blend.

| 3 parts yarrow tincture | 1 part shepherd's purse *(Capsella bursa-pastoris)* tincture | 1 part nettle tincture |

1 Blend and bottle the tinctures, label, and add to your kit.

2 Give 30 to 60 drops every 15 minutes until some improvement is obvious, and then begin to back off to every 30 minutes, then to every hour, and then to 3 to 6 times daily, providing that signs of improvement are clear.

🌱 MIGRAINE RELIEF 🌱

Do you need a migraine remedy in your kit? Maybe, maybe not. But if you or someone in your family routinely gets migraines, then you absolutely do. Migraines are debilitating and can leave a person in pain, nauseous, and sensitive to light for several days in a row. Try these remedies now when the next migraine hits to see which works best. Migraines can be at the base of the head or behind an eye. They tend to happen on only one side of the head, and usually the same side each time. Other types of headaches can be brought on by dehydration, stress, and sinus pressure.

Feverfew *(Tanacetum parthenium)*. Take this classic herbal migraine and headache remedy by either tincture or capsule. It may not be the best option for anyone allergic to ragweed as they are from the same plant family and may trigger an allergic reaction.

Peppermint. At the first sign of a migraine, take peppermint tea or apply a drop of peppermint essential oil to each temple. Be aware that many people cannot handle peppermint essential oil directly on the skin and must use a carrier oil such as grapeseed oil.

Personally, peppermint essential oil used directly on my temples doesn't irritate me. That does not mean it's safe to use it that way. Every person is different. Use a carrier oil if necessary. Try adding a drop to the palms, rubbing them together, cupping them over the nose, and inhaling. If peppermint oil is still too irritating, try lavender essential oil instead. Most people tolerate lavender well, although it doesn't help my headaches as well as peppermint.

Codonopsis. Take by tincture. It is safe for use by children and during pregnancy.

☙ NAUSEA/MOTION SICKNESS ☙

I would get carsick on long trips when I was young, and sometimes it happens to me even now. Nausea is a pretty common symptom, especially for children and during pregnancy. Let's say something has happened, and you have decided it's time to bug out before things get worse, especially if one of your concerns is traffic from your primary location to your bugout. You need to leave before the highways and secondary routes become parking lots.

Unfortunately, a child or a pregnant woman in your group is nauseous.

Sometimes, you can't do anything but pull over and let nature take its course. Other times, there are tips and tricks, as well as some herbal help to avoid becoming nauseous or to nip nausea in the bud before it gets out of hand.

Sitting in the front may not be safest place, but it does naturally cause people to look straight ahead instead of out the side windows. This can help with car sickness. The noise of the vehicle and the tires on the road can irritate the inner ear and cause nausea as well. Having the radio on may distract you from your outside environment, but it can cut down on car sickness. And as much as I don't care for kids being dependent on electronic entertainment, having an MP3 player with earbuds can help without distracting the driver. A DVD player with headphones is even better. It keeps the focus away from the windows, blocks out road noise, and doesn't take away from the driver's situational awareness.

As for herbs, having a thermos of peppermint, chamomile, or ginger tea prepared ahead for the ride is a good idea. By the time car sickness sets in, it's probably at a good temperature to drink. Candied ginger is a convenient way to keep ginger in your first aid kit without spoiling.

❦ PAIN RELIEF SALVE ❦

Thankfully, most injuries are not nearly so dramatic or serious as gunshot wounds, deep lacerations, or internal bleeding. I spent years caring for non-life-threatening pain in my massage practice. Muscle injuries, spasms, poor body alignment, hip problems, and a host of painful conditions are far more common injuries that, at best, will slow you down and, at worst, leave you vulnerable to some other threat.

One of my favorite remedies for injured muscles and joints is this warming pain relief salve when heat is appropriate. (Heat is not appropriate for acute injuries; use ice immediately after an injury.) Cayenne is loaded with capsaicin, which helps to create a warming sensation in the layers of tissue as it sinks into the skin. It brings the blood to the injured site, and with the blood comes more oxygen and nourishment. Capsaicin also numbs the nerve endings, helping to alleviate the sensation of pain.

This salve also includes St. John's wort infused oil. While St. John's wort can be used dry in capsules and to make a tincture, the flowers must be used fresh to get a decent infused oil. The oil can then be used throughout the year. St. John's wort nourishes the nervous system, helping the body recover from anxiety and nerve pain. I've found it immensely helpful for back pain, especially low back pain, as well as sciatica.

Arnica and goldenrod both add pain-relieving properties. My observation from using variations of this salve is that arnica seems to alleviate discomfort more in the joints and structures, whereas goldenrod seems to help more with discomforts in the muscles, tendons, ligaments, and connective tissues.

Sunflower oil	⅛ cup arnica infused oil	Optional: 48 drops clove essential oil (omit for sensitive skin)
½ cup cayenne infused oil	⅛ cup goldenrod infused oil	
¼ cup St. John's wort infused oil	1 tablespoon beeswax	

1   Make individual infused oils of the above herbs in sunflower oil. Each is so useful for multiple recipes that it's far better to make them separately and then mix as needed. Sunflower oil is lighter than olive oil and absorbs into the skin a little easier. You could use olive oil if you wanted to make a massage oil instead of a salve.

2   This salve requires 1 cup of total oil. I've indicated my preferred amounts of infused oils, including the ones infused from St. John's wort, arnica, and goldenrod flowers. Feel free to adjust as desired.

3   Melt the beeswax into the infused oils in a double boiler on low heat. Do not cook the oils. Using only 1 tablespoon of beeswax will allow the salve to penetrate the skin more easily.

4   After the wax has completely melted, remove from the heat. You now have a perfectly effective salve. However, if you wish to include the essential oil, this is the time to do so.

5   If you choose to add an essential oil, clove or one of your own selections, add it directly to your containers, pour the salve over the oil, and cap immediately. Label the containers, and put one in your kit.

❦ PAIN TINCTURE: MAJOR ❦

I cannot take an ounce of credit for this wonderful combination of herbs. It came from the individual writings and efforts of two herbalists, Kerry Bone and Kiva Rose. Kerry Bone has a product in a pill form that includes California poppy, corydalis, and Jamaican dogwood bark.

Then I found a variation of this combination on Kiva Rose's blog. While both herbalists have a poppy as the primary ingredient, Kiva Rose uses Mexican poppy *(Eschscholzia californica mexicana)*. She combines these herbs in tincture form instead of a pill, which I prefer because the herbs will be absorbed faster into the system with the assistance of the alcohol. The faster you can relieve the pain, the better. She also uses more corydalis than Jamaican dogwood in her blend, whereas Kerry Bone uses more Jamaican dogwood than corydalis.

I got to test this tincture for the first time when my husband's back was injured. I had California poppy, corydalis, and Jamaican dogwood tinctures on hand, so I blended them together. Shortly after taking it, my husband was fast asleep. The herbs are known to cause drowsiness, but he had also been awake for two nights without sleep due to the pain. I've since taken it myself after a bad fall, and used it in my practice. Apply caution as the treatment does induce drowsiness.

3 parts California poppy	2 parts corydalis *(Corydalis yanhusuo)*	1 part Jamaican dogwood *(Piscidia piscipula)*

1   Mix the above tinctures, or tincture the above proportions of herbs.

2   Bottle and label.

3   Take 20 to 30 drops as needed.

I would try dosing every 20 minutes at first, perhaps only for the first hour, and then as needed after that. Pay attention to the length of intervals between necessary doses. As the injury heals, you will want to spread these doses out more. Do not operate vehicles or heavy machinery when taking this remedy. Of course, if you have severe pain, you shouldn't be out doing that anyway. Stay home and rest up! This remedy is not for pregnant women.

☙ PAIN TINCTURE: ☙ MINOR/MODERATE

White willow tincture is safe and effective in relieving mild to moderate pain, providing there is no allergy to aspirin and, if for a child, no fever present. While there is no evidence that the natural salicin in white willow bark causes the same allergic reaction as the synthetic version found in aspirin, it's better to err on the side of caution.

This caution holds true also for the warning against aspirin during an infection when giving to children. Although there is no evidence that herbs with salicin may cause Reye's syndrome the way synthetic aspirin does, unfortunately there has not been a study in this area. It's prudent to apply the same warnings from aspirin to herbs that contain natural salicin.

Keeping these cautions in mind, I like to try white willow first for all types of aches and pains, including headaches, sprains, and arthritis. I would describe it as more effective and longer lasting than aspirin, and it doesn't upset my stomach, which is something that synthetic aspirin does.

When dealing with a severe sprain, between my instructions and my husband's patient willingness to learn how to do the actual crafting, I instructed him to blend the following tinctures of herbs, with 1 ounce equal to 1 "part," to help reduce the pain and inflammation.

3 parts white willow bark	1 part corydalis yanhusuo
2 parts black cohosh	1 part ginger

If an ingredient is not appropriate for you, leave it out. Otherwise, consider some of the topical salves for pain in this chapter.

☙ POISON IVY/POISON OAK SALVE ☙

When people describe plants and herbs as slow and gentle, they have probably never had an encounter with poison ivy, poison oak, or poison sumac and experienced the itchy rash. Try this salve if you have the unfortunate experience to encounter one of these plants. Jewel weed (one of those extra herbs I've squeezed in here) needs a lighter oil than olive oil, because it doesn't absorb very well.

1 ounce sunflower oil	1 ounce grindelia	1 tablespoon beeswax
1 ounce jewel weed (impatiens)	1 ounce plantain	48 drops tea tree oil

1   Infuse jewel weed (use the whole plant, but break or cut the stems as much as possible), grindelia, and plantain into the sunflower oil.

2 Melt the beeswax into 1 cup of the infused oil.

3 Remove from the heat, and let cool slightly.

4 Add tea tree to each jar or tin equal to 2% of the container. If you are using a 2-ounce jar or tin, that is about 20 to 25 drops (2% of 2 ounces is a little over 1 ml, and 1 ml is 20 drops).

5 Label the containers, add one to your kit, and store the rest.

🐝 POISON IVY/POISON OAK SPRAY 🐝

If you prefer to spray on relief, give this a try. Spray as needed.

16 fluid ounces witch hazel	**3 ounces (by weight) grindelia**	**Optional: 96 drops total of any combination of lavender, peppermint, or tea tree essential oils**
3 ounces (by weight) jewel weed		

1 If you have just jewel weed or just grindelia, go ahead and use 6 ounces of the single herb. It will still work.

2 Add herbs to a quart mason jar, and cover with witch hazel.

3 Allow to steep for 4 to 6 weeks, then strain out the herbs.

4 If desired, add essential oils to the spray bottle.

5 Pour in liquid, and label the spray bottle. Place in your kit, and store the rest.

🐝 RESPIRATORY INFECTION TEA 🐝

This is one of my favorite remedies for a respiratory infection that grips the chest. I like to call it "herbal tussin tea."

2 cups hyssop flowers	**1½ cups slippery elm root**	**½ cup coltsfoot (Tussilago farfara), aerial parts**
1½ cups mullein leaves	**1 cup elecampagne root**	

½ cup marshmallow root	½ cup spearmint leaves	½ cup licorice root
		½ cup thyme leaves
	½ cup whole cloves	

1. Blend these ingredients together.

2. Transfer to a jar or tin, label, and put in your kit. Store the rest in either a mason jar or a Mylar bag with oxygen absorbers.

3. Prepare this tea as an infusion. While there are roots and tough plant parts in it, enough of their medicine comes through.

4. Take 4 to 6 cups daily.

🐍 SNAKE- AND SPIDER-BITE CARE 🐍

Even if you live somewhere that naturally lacks venomous snakes and spiders, that doesn't mean they aren't out there. Unfortunately, some people think keeping venomous creatures for their private collection is a good idea.

In my area, we have a population of timber rattlesnakes, northern copperheads, and northern black widow spiders. Even though snakes are not commonly seen in our small city, one afternoon I spotted something on top of a shrub while on my way into my old apartment building. At first I couldn't quite make out what it was. The color seemed to blend into the bush, and it looked something like a garden hose coiled up. It would have been a very odd place for maintenance to leave a garden hose. As I walked closer to my door, I saw a head come up, and I froze in place.

Although I would love to tell an exciting tale about a harrowing encounter I was lucky enough to survive, what I actually encountered was a large, nonvenomous garter snake basking in the sun. However, it spooked me enough to start looking into which creatures in our area are venomous.

Of course, the remedy always given for venom is antivenom. Well, I don't have a laboratory in my basement, and my herbal workspace is about as mad scientist as I get. So, antivenom isn't going to work in a situation where hospitals and medical interventions are out of the question.

Checking around first aid supplies and camping supply shops, I found the Sawyer Extractor Pump, which is advertised as using suction to draw out venom. While I understand the concept and I had some hope for it, I found that scientific studies of the pump were less than impressive. It is apparently capable of sucking out some bloody fluid but doesn't do a good job of extracting venom. One study found it extracted no venom at all.[15]

Here are some general guidelines for venomous bites:

If you are still in the vicinity of where the bite happened, calmly check for signs of the snake (or spider, scorpion, or other creature) and move to safety if necessary. This may mean carrying the bite victim out of the area. Walking increases circulation, and you don't want to encourage the venom to spread.

Keep the person calm. Ask if you may help. Talk to him or her about each step in your evaluation and proposed treatment. Speaking slowly and deliberately is helpful in keeping a person calm.

Examine the bite. First, make sure there is no venom on the surface of the skin. If there is, make sure not to come in contact yourself. Use some kind of barrier, such as protective gloves, and use either water and soap, or alcohol-soaked pads from your kit, to thoroughly wipe away the venom. Take care when disposing of anything that may have come in contact with the venom so no one else accidentally is exposed.

Then check for swelling and discoloration. If there is discoloration, mark it with a pen, and come back to that spot periodically over the next few hours to see if the damage has spread.

If possible, keep the site of the bite lower than the heart, and have the bitten person stay off his or her feet. More movement equals more circulation, and more circulation of the venom.

Other ways to draw out the toxin include activated charcoal, bentonite clay, plantain, or any of the ingredients from the drawing salve on page 154.

---

15   Michael B. Alberts et al., "Suction for Venomous Snakebite: A Study of 'Mock Venom' Extraction in a Human Model," *Annals of Emergency Medicine* 43, no. 2 (2003): 181–86.

The charcoal or clay may not actually be reaching the venom, depending on the size of the puncture wound from the snake's teeth, which can often be more like needles than tissue-ripping fangs. Drawing agents are still worth a try, as activated charcoal is capable of drawing out brown recluse venom. Just be aware that such drawing agents are not foolproof.

In addition to applying drawing herbs topically, you may find that a blend of tinctures helps. Much depends on the type of snake bite, the health and size of the person, and a host of other factors. 80% of the world's population uses herbal medicine, so some herbs are known for treating snakebite, and some have studies to support that use.16 This tincture includes herbs with traditional use in snakebites, either to counter the venom, lower edema, or stimulate the body's cleansing processes.

3 parts sida tincture	3 parts turmeric tincture	1 part milk thistle tincture
3 parts echinacea tincture	2 parts black cohosh tincture	1 part burdock tincture

Additionally, give encapsulated andrographis, size 00 capsules, approximately 700 mg (not part of tincture).

1. Blend the single tinctures or make a tincture of the herbs in the above proportions.

2. Bottle and label. Add one to your kit, and store the rest.

3. Prepare capsules from powdered andrographis (exceedingly bitter, take encapsulated). Give tincture frequently, every 30 to 60 minutes if bite radius is spreading. Give 2 capsules every hour if bite radius is spreading.

4. Adjust dosing based on observations. If bite radius is not spreading, slow down tincture and capsules to every 3 hours.

There are many factors in whether or not a snake or spider bite becomes fatal. This is an area of natural medicine that I hope sees far more research. Thankfully, most bites do not have enough venom to be fatal. It is often our fear, racing heart, and panic that help to circulate and spread the

16   Y.K. Gupta and S.S. Peshin, "Do Herbal Medicines Have Potential for Managing Snake Bite Envenomation?" *Toxicology International* 19, no. 2 (2012): 89–99.

venom through the body. The best thing to do when there is no hospital or emergency care available is to get still, get as comfortable as possible, use the natural remedies you have, and do your best to wait it out as calmly as possible.

🐝 SNAKEBITE AND TOXIN 🐝 DRAWING SALVE

Sometimes, you need to draw a toxin, a venom, or even a splinter out of tissue. There are certain types of bites that I handle differently, but I carry this as a general, all-purpose drawing salve.

1 part olive oil	1 part comfrey	2 tablespoons bentonite clay
1 part plantain leaves	1 tablespoon beeswax	
1 part mullein leaves	2 tablespoons activated charcoal powder	2 tablespoons honey (optional)
1 part calendula flowers		

1   Make an infused oil of equal amounts of plantain, mullein, calendula, and comfrey in olive oil.

2   Melt the beeswax into the oil in a double boiler on low heat. Do not cook the oil.

3   When the wax has melted completely, remove from the heat and transfer the oil and wax to a mixing bowl.

4   Add the activated charcoal and bentonite. Stir to incorporate.

5   The salve will begin to cool. You can either pour the salve as is into containers, or you can add honey.

6   Adding honey is a little tricky, since you don't want to cook raw honey, but you need the salve warm enough to be liquid. Look for a point where the salve is cooling a little on the sides but is still liquid in the middle, but barely so. Add 2 tablespoons of warm, runny honey. Either stir the honey in, or if the salve has cooled

off too much or the honey wasn't warm enough, you can force the honey to blend with an immersion blender.

7 Scoop the salve into jars or tins, smooth the top with a spatula, and wipe the edges of the containers clean.

8 Label the containers, add one to your kit, and store the rest.

❧ SORE THROAT SPRAY ❧

Here is the perfect example of how berberine and echinacea can work together harmoniously in a throat spray. If you can, gargle with saltwater gargle first, and then spray as needed to numb the throat.

2 fluid ounces spilanthes tincture

2 fluid ounces *Echinacea angustifolia* tincture

2 fluid ounces berberine tincture (type local to you)

1 tablespoon honey

1 tablespoon lemon juice

2 to 5 drops peppermint essential oil

1 Mix the tinctures together, and then blend in the honey and lemon juice. You should have a total of 8 fluid ounces.

2 Add peppermint essential oil for flavor.

3 Pour into two 4-ounce spray bottles, and label them. Put one in your kit, and store the other.

❧ SPRAINS AND BRUISES ❧ SALVE/POULTICE

Contusions, a.k.a. bruises, are injuries to blood vessels that show up at the surface of the skin as dark areas. They can be small or large, and a faint dark color or deep blue. The longer it takes a bruise to come to the surface, the deeper the wound. Contusions can be signs of other injury below the skin, especially when accompanied by pain and inflammation. This type of injury may be a strain, sprain, or a fracture that needs further care.

I keep a blend of the herbs for this treatment in a jar to be used as a compress. I also use these herbs in a salve in case there just isn't the option to set up a compress. For example, if I notice a bruise on my son (who knows what he banged into) but he's otherwise fine, I apply the herbs as a salve.

If someone sprained an ankle and we had to leave the area quickly, I would slather this salve on, tape it up, and get out of there. Later on, I would apply the herbs in a poultice. If the situation were less urgent, I would take the time to get the person off his or her feet, get the foot elevated, and make a poultice.

Instead of regular flour, the lavender powder in this recipe adds a nice dimension to the remedy, calming the injured person. You could also get lavender into the salve either through infused oil or by adding lavender essential oil at the end, but I haven't found that lavender oil makes as much of a difference to the salve as lavender powder does to a poultice.

Olive oil (for salve)	Goldenrod flowers	Beeswax (for salve)
Comfrey leaves	Self-heal *(Prunella vulgaris)*	Lavender flower powder (for poultice)
Arnica flowers		

FOR SALVE

1 Make an infused oil of equal portions of herbs and olive oil.

2 Melt 2 tablespoons of beeswax into 1 cup of the infused oil in a double boiler on low heat to avoid cooking the oil.

3 Strain the herbs, and pour the liquid into jars or tins.

4 Allow to cool, and label the containers.

5 Add one to your kit, and store the rest.

FOR POULTICE

1 Mix equal portions of well-chopped herbs, except the lavender powder (kept in a separate jar), in a large mixing bowl. I usually use ½ cup as a portion.

2 Fill a jar with herbs for your kit, and store the rest in mason jars or Mylar bags with oxygen absorbers until needed.

3   Add the herbs, except the lavender powder, to a pot and cover with clean water. Gently warm the water for no more than 5 minutes, and remove from heat.

4   Add the lavender powder to thicken the poultice, and make a paste.

5   This blend contains arnica, which should be used only on closed wounds. Also, arnica is not for use during pregnancy. It is, however, a wonderful, well-researched pain reliever. If you want to omit the arnica, go ahead.

Comfrey comes with a generic warning not to use during pregnancy because of the presence of alkaloid pyrrolizidine alkalide (PA; see Comfrey page 70). However, this is one of those "use your common sense" moments. I would not drink comfrey root tea while pregnant. However, for short-term, topical use on a bad sprain, I would use the leaves, which have less PA, and be comfortable with that choice. I haven't seen anything that demonstrates a clear risk during pregnancy for that type of application. Do some additional reading on comfrey, and come to your own conclusion.

🍄 STRESS, ANXIETY, AND 🍄 TRAUMATIC EVENTS

Clearly, if a worst-case scenario occurs, there are going to be emotionally distressed people who will see and experience things they never imagined. Ideally, access to professional therapists after a major trauma would be great. Herbalists are not that. However, we as individuals need to have a plan to help those in distress, including ourselves.

There are many nerve-calming herbs, known as nervines. Often, simply drinking some tea made from oats, chamomile, and lemon balm is sufficient for me to come back to center when I'm being pulled in a thousand different directions between work, family, the temper tantrums of small children, household chores and errands, homeschooling, podcasting, writing, prepping, and who knows what else. And those are still everyday stresses. They are not major traumas.

A tincture can enhance the calming tea. When you make your tea of oats, chamomile, and lemon balm, add 30 to 60 drops of valerian or American skullcap tincture while the herbs are steeping. I find it's a better-tasting way to take those tinctures anyway.

You may need several options, as not all herbs work the same on all people. Do not discount the value of a cup of tea to calm and steady a person. There is something very soothing and grounding about sitting down with a hot cup of herbal brew, inhaling the steam, and drinking it like some magical relaxation potion. Here are some options I find very relaxing:

+ Valerian tincture

+ Skullcap tincture

+ Rose petal infused honey, by the spoonful as needed

+ Kava kava pastilles

+ Rhodiola tincture

+ Any combination of the above

To make the kava kava pastilles: Mix kava kava powder with honey by adding the honey a little at a time and mixing thoroughly. Stop adding honey when the mixture is the consistency of dough and holds its shape. Roll into little balls between your fingers, press flat, and allow to air-dry.

❦ URINARY TRACT INFECTION ❦ TINCTURE AND TEA

When people are under stress, do not drink enough water, and have no access to hygienic conditions, urinary tract infections (UTI) can develop. They are usually caused by E. coli, but can also be caused and aggravated by sexual intercourse. Make each tincture individually, and then blend and bottle for your kit.

Marshmallow root does not tincture well. Instead, make a tea from a cold infusion of the root and milky oat tops. The demulcent herbs helps to soothe irritated tissues.

TINCTURE BLEND

1 part bilberry tincture

1 part berberine tincture (type local to you)

1 part juniper berry tincture

1 part dandelion root tincture

1 part corn silk tincture (collect silk when shucking corn)

1 part nettle seed tincture

1 Blend the tinctures together.

2 Bottle, label, and add to your kit.

3 Take a standard 30 to 60 drop dose, 3 to 6 times per day, until symptoms are gone.

TEA BLEND

1 cup marshmallow root

½ cup milky oat tops

1 In a quart mason jar, add the marshmallow root and milky oat tops.

2 Fill to the top with room-temperature clean water.

3 Allow to sit at room temperature for at least 4 hours, or up to 12 hours.

4 Strain and drink throughout the day. Be sure to drink water and cranberry juice as well.

❦ WOUND, BURN, OR ❦ "SHTF" HONEY

There really is nothing like raw honey for a wound or a burn. You don't even have to do anything to it for it to be ideal first aid for a serious cut, puncture, or even full-thickness burn. And while you don't have to do anything to raw honey for it to heal a wound and prevent infection, you can infuse it with herbs to add additional layers of healing properties.

Apply honey after you stop the bleeding and clean out the wound. You don't want to dilute the honey, and you don't want to trap dirt or particulates in the wound when it's healing.

Approximately 2 pounds (32 ounces) raw honey, with some left over

1 part St. John's wort flowers

1 part lavender flowers

1 part sida aerial parts

1 part plantain

1. Fill a mason jar about three-quarters full with the herbs.

2. Fill to the top with the raw honey, allowing the honey to settle and adding more until the jar is filled. Use a plastic knife to get rid of any air pockets. Secure tightly with a lid to keep out any moisture.

3. Allow the honey to infuse for 6 weeks, or use a slow cooker. Place the mason jar in a slow cooker, and fill the pot up to one-quarter full with water. Allow to steep on low for 2 hours, then turn the slow cooker off. Let the jar sit in the slow cooker until it is cool. If your slow cooker has a warm setting, allow it to continue steeping for 4 to 6 hours. Just be very careful not to let the honey get above 115°F to avoid cooking off the enzymes in the honey. Better yet, keep it under 110°F.

4. While the honey is warm and runny, strain out the herbs.

5. Bottle, allow to cool, and label.

6. Add the bottle to your kit, and store any extra.

❦ WOUND CARE TINCTURE ❦

This tincture can be applied externally to stop bleeding, provide a bit of numbing, and cut down on infection. I make each tincture separately based on the information in Chapter 4, Materia Medica, and blend them.

4 parts yarrow tincture (controls the flow of blood)

2 parts echinacea tincture (fights infections, somewhat numbing)

1 part spilanthes tincture (fights infection, somewhat numbing)

1 part berberine tincture, type local to you (fights infection)

1   Apply by the capful (common with HDPE bottles) or dropperful
     (pipettes are more common for glass) directly to the wound every
     15 minutes while also applying pressure until the bleeding has
     stopped.

2   Pour into a bottle for your first aid/trauma kit, and store the rest
     in a bottle for storage or home use. Label and add to your kit and
     supplies.

❦ WOUND POWDER: ❦ ANTIBACTERIAL

Another option for wounds is an antibacterial wound powder that can
help stop bleeding and prevent infection. The powder will have to be
cleaned out carefully, as it may clump, although removing it may cause the
wound to start bleeding again. However, it does a good job of helping the
tissues stay healthy as they heal.

| 1 part yarrow flowers | 1 part marshmallow root | 1 part usnea |
| | | 1 part kaolin clay |

1   Dry and powder the herbs.

2   Blend equal amounts of each herb and the clay, and keep in a jar
     or bottle that will allow you to shake out the powder, preferably
     with one hand. This will allow you to continue to apply pressure
     with the other hand.

3   Label the container, and add it to your kit.

❦ WOUND WASH ❦

This wash has multiple uses, which is important in a first aid kit. I use the
wash for both wounds and burns. My kit contains two bottles: a 4-ounce
spray bottle and a 16-ounce squeeze bottle. I used the squeeze bottle to
flush a wound, and the spray bottle on minor abrasions as well as sunburn.
For a more serious burn on the hand when there isn't any clean water to
cool the burn, I would empty the larger bottle into a basin and soak the

hand. Note that the herbs in the following list are measured by weight and the witch hazel by volume.

16 ounces witch hazel extract

1 ounce plantain leaves

1 ounce berberine (type local to you)

1 ounce thyme leaves

1 Infuse equal amounts of thyme, plantain, and berberine into witch hazel, and let soak for 4 to 6 weeks.

2 Strain out the herbs, and bottle the liquid.

3 Label the bottle, and add to your kit.

CHAPTER 6

EVERYDAY NATURAL MEDICINE

Let food be thy medicine and medicine be thy food.
—Hippocrates

Walking is man's best medicine.
—Hippocrates

In addition to a first aid plan, everyone needs a plan for preventive care, chronic illness, and common infections such as cold and flu. The key to being prepared lies in preventive care. By creating health, you reduce the instance of illness. Many chronic diseases are related to lifestyle. By changing habits, it's possible to eliminate much of the heart disease, hypertension, obesity, and diabetes, and certain cancers common in our modern society. Preventive care means taking a proactive stance about health and taking steps to improve it. This begins with nutrient-dense foods, clean water, clean air, and plenty of movement.

In addition to discussing nutritional concerns and preventive care, this chapter looks at herbal strategies to fill the gap when diet and lifestyle are not enough. I have included natural recipes to help cope with some of the most common illnesses when preventive care falls short. Most of us either are on some kind of maintenance drug or know someone who is. If access to pharmacies is cut off, many people will be without their blood pressure, asthma, allergy, arthritis, and cholesterol medications, and those circumstances require a plan B.

This chapter introduces women's natural medicine, an important topic for everyday natural medicine as well as long-term preparedness. There is so much information to consider about the unique health concerns of women that it could easily be a book all on its own. In this chapter, I briefly touch on the most common concerns that women face, including PMS, birth control, pregnancy, and menopause.

NUTRITIONAL SYRUPS

Good health starts with good nutrition. Consider the fact that magnesium is involved in more than 300 functions in the body. Then consider how modern agricultural practices have depleted magnesium from the soil. If it's not in the soil, then it's not in the food. Suddenly, the reason for many of our chronic states of unhealth become clear. And that's just one nutrient! I am not a fan of the U.S. government's food guidelines, as I don't think the recommended daily allowances (RDA) of nutrients are high enough to maintain health.

Although lacking in calories, many herbs are nutritionally dense. Stinging nettle is so nutritionally dense that I consider it a superfood. It contains vitamins A, C, D, E, and K; bioflavonoids; B vitamins such as thiamin, riboflavin, niacin, and B6 folate; and choline. Nettle is rich in minerals, such as calcium, magnesium, iron, zinc, selenium, boron, iodine, copper, and chromium. Finally, nettle is high in chlorophyll, is very useful if you have been exposed to radiation, addresses pancreatitis, and helps in healing wounds.

Also of note, nettle is a complete protein with 16 essential amino acids. Its amino acid profile is similar to that of eggs. Furthermore, 40% of the dried leaf is protein. Fresh, the leaf contains more water but is approximately 22% to 25% protein. To put this into grams instead of percentages, there are 2.4 grams of protein in 1 cup of nettle, compared with 1 gram of protein in 1 cup of boiled beans.

I'm not suggesting that anyone stop eating meat in favor of nettle, but nettle can supplement protein intake during lean times. The government recommends that we eat about 50 grams of protein per day. It would take 20 cups of nettle to get the full day's requirement for protein. That is a lot of nettle! The 2.4 grams mentioned above is only about 4% of the daily recommendation. In contrast, 1 egg contains much more protein at 6 grams, or 12% of the daily recommendation.

Harvesting nettle can be tricky because of the sting (which goes away upon drying or cooking), so use gloves or tongs, or fold the leaves to avoid coming in contact with the stinging hairs underneath. Once the plant has finished growing, you can make the stems into cordage. The stinging nature of nettle means it can be used as part of a security hedge. The sting feels like a less intense bee sting, but to move through an entire patch of nettle is quite unpleasant without proper protection.

Nettle is included in the Nutritional Syrup recipe under Fracture and Broken Bones Poultice (page 141). You can vary the recipe by using different herbs and sweeteners. The recipe calls for molasses, but feel free to use maple syrup, birch syrup, or honey instead. Each sweetener has some nutritional benefits.

Lately, I have been using yacon syrup. I want to experiment with growing yacon tubers, which look very much like sweet potatoes. The tuber produces a syrup from the cooked-down juice that's similar in texture and appearance to molasses, but tastes more like caramel. Initial studies have shown yacon syrup to have a lower impact on blood sugar because of its high fiber content. And who wouldn't want medicine or nutritional supplements to taste like caramel?

Nutritional syrups can be customized for women or men, pregnancy, chronic conditions, and so on. Customizing your nutritional syrup allows you to take one combined remedy instead of multiple separate remedies. This combination approach makes it easy for people to follow through.

Syrups have a limited shelf life. They may last a couple of days on the counter, depending on room temperature and water content. In the refrigerator, I've seen syrups last anywhere from a few weeks to a few months. I store the dry ingredients and sweeteners separately, and make my nutritional syrups in small batches. If you have a storage freezer, you could freeze large amounts of syrup, but if your freezer lost power or stopped working, then you would lose everything in it.

Rather than the basic recipe for Nutritional Syrup included in the previous chapter, this is the version I take daily, along with my version of fire cider tonic. I take this syrup and fire cider tonic 3 times daily, about 30 minutes before each meal. It's easier for me to remember to take them both by sticking to a schedule. Otherwise, take a nutritional syrup like this anywhere between 2 and 6 times daily, depending on your body's needs. If you've been ill, take more. A child can take less.

❦ CAT'S FAVORITE ❦ NUTRITIONAL SYRUP

½ cup dandelion root

¼ cup burdock

¼ cup yellow dock

1 part nettle leaves

1 part alfalfa

1 part horsetail

1 part red raspberry leaves

1 part parsley

1 part rose hips

1 part oatstraw

Yacon syrup or honey

1   Make a double decoction of the dandelion, burdock, and yellow dock in 4 cups of water. I use these herbs not for their function as bitters, but for their minerals. After straining the herbs, you should have approximately 1 cup of liquid.

2   While the double decoction is reducing, blend equal parts of nettle, alfalfa, horsetail, red raspberry, parsley, rose hips, and oatstraw.

3   While the strained double decoction is still hot (reheat if necessary), add ½ cup of the blended herbs to the hot liquid to steep, covered, for 30 minutes.

4   Strain the herbs and pour the liquid into a 16-ounce (2-cup) bottle. It should be less than half full. Add enough yacon syrup to bring the total volume to 16 ounces. Cap the bottle, and shake vigorously to mix.

If using honey instead of yacon, make sure the liquid is warm, around 90°F. This will help the honey blend into the syrup more easily.

One problem remains: Fat-soluble vitamins are missing from a water extraction. However, nettle can be made into a soup with a cream base or into pesto. Top with some pumpkin seeds and the result is nearly perfect nutrition. Many recipes for soup made from fresh or dried nettle are available online.

BOOSTING THE IMMUNE SYSTEM

I have a lot of favorites when it comes to natural medicine. Who can blame me? There's a lot to love. Fire cider ranks as a favorite among favorites. Herbalist Rosemary Gladstar, who has generously shared her recipe through workshops, books, and YouTube, has made this traditional immunity-boosting remedy famous.

Just about every herbalist who makes this traditional health tonic has put his or her own spin on it. My own version has seen several adaptations, and will probably see more as I tinker with it.

Fire cider is an oxymel, an herbal vinegar mixed with honey. I use raw apple cider vinegar and raw honey. As its name implies, fire cider is spicy. Its kick comes from plenty of cayenne and horseradish, with a warming sensation from fresh ginger. The garlic tends to mellow as it steeps in the vinegar, as does the onion. The flavor is just a bit different every time, depending on how hot the cayenne and horseradish are, how fresh the ginger is, and how much of each ingredient ends up steeping in the vinegar. Making this remedy is more like cooking, where you are free to adjust amounts, than it is like baking, where you must carefully measure ingredients.

Fire cider isn't just hot. It's also pungent, sour, and intense. That might not sound tempting at first, but once you start taking it, it's hard to stop. I take mine by the ounce, in 2 ounces of apple juice. You can take it straight if you really like strong flavors.

❦ TRADITIONAL FIRE CIDER ❦

Onion

Garlic

Horseradish

Cayenne

Ginger root

Raw apple cider vinegar

Honey

1   There are no specified amounts of each ingredient. Experiment until you arrive at a blend you like.

2 Layer the onion, garlic, horseradish, cayenne, and ginger in a quart or larger mason jar. Fill the jar three-quarters full. The herbs will expand as they absorb some of the vinegar.

3 Pour enough apple cider vinegar to cover all the ingredients. Wait a few minutes to let the vinegar work its way down and into the jar, filling all the nooks and crannies where air bubbles are hiding. Run a butter knife down the sides to release any trapped air and get the vinegar into all the spaces.

4 Top off with more apple cider vinegar, and cap.

5 Allow to steep for 2 to 4 weeks.

6 Strain out all the ingredients, and reserve the liquid.

7 Measure the liquid, and add one-half the volume in honey. For example, add 1 cup of honey to 2 cups of infused vinegar. However, feel free to adjust the amount of honey to your taste.

In my version, I add turmeric, astragalus, Siberian ginseng, lemon juice, and hawthorn berries. I have at other times included thyme, rosemary, sage, lemon zest, and orange zest. I have seen some herbalists include rose hips, blueberries, and schisandra berries.

Many people take fire cider as an immune tonic and to ward off colds and flu. Sometimes, the full extent of a remedy's benefits cannot be understood if the person taking the remedy is already in a good state of health. Give the same remedy to someone who is in a state of unhealth, and suddenly the remedy is a miracle potion.

I have worked with some very unhealthy people with multiple diagnoses of vague syndromes, such as fatigue, general achiness, weight gain, weight loss, headaches, brain "fog," and a general sense of being unwell. I often give them variations of fire cider made with their general complaints in mind. Often, I also suggest a nutritional syrup, some digestive bitters, and fermented foods (or at least a probiotic supplement).

I have had people tell me that fire cider helped reduce some of their aches and pains, as well as sinus inflammation. I'm not surprised, as it is loaded with anti-inflammatory ingredients. I've had others confess that their bowel movements became easier and were "cleaner" since they started taking fire cider daily—not in a sudden, harsh laxative way, but in a gentle, subtle shift.

SUGAR AND SICKNESS

If there is one culinary culprit more responsible for illness than sugar, I don't know what it is. High sugar consumption is responsible for most obesity, high blood pressure, type 2 diabetes, hypoglycemia, polycystic ovarian syndrome (PCOS), elevated cholesterol, and lower immune response. One of the single best things you can do for your health is cut back on sugar.

Sugar isn't just the obvious white crystals. It is in our grains, alcohol, and starchy vegetables. Marketing magicians have been hard at work for decades convincing us that whole grains are good for us. There really isn't much difference between a slice of white bread with 1 gram of dietary fiber and a slice of whole wheat bread with 2 grams of dietary fiber. The reality is that whole grains have only a small amount more nutrition, just a little more fiber, and about the same impact on blood glucose as processed white rice, white wheat, and other white grains. When the body breaks down the grains, processed or whole, there is very little fiber to slow down the impact on blood sugar.

This doesn't mean you should never eat grains. I have a lot of oatmeal in my food storage. Just be aware that high sugar consumption is at the root of cardiovascular disease,[17] hypoglycemia, type 2 diabetes, metabolic syndrome, candida, and obesity. If you have any of these issues, you may be better served by replacing grain with vegetables as your primary source of carbohydrates, at least for a while. Vegetables really do have a lot of fiber. You might want to take that one step further and go with fermented veggies to promote healthy gut flora. Lacto-fermentation also makes the nutrients in foods more bioavailable and helps to extend their shelf life.

---

17 Quanhe Yang et al., "Added Sugar Intake and Cardiovascular Diseases Mortality Among US Adults," *JAMA Internal Medicine* 174, no. 4 (2014): 516–24.

With brain fog clearing, less achiness, and easier elimination, people move more and sleep better. Little by little, over time, that general malaise and sense of being unwell lift, and many of the odd symptoms that seemingly have no cause just fade away. At this point, any symptoms remaining get individual attention. But the subtle changes, the daily ritual of taking homemade medicine, and the tonic, anti-inflammatory, and immune-boosting herbs in the menstruum of raw apple cider vinegar with its liver-protective and blood sugar–modulating properties—all of this can have a profound effect on people who are wildly out of balance.

I have also found fire cider very useful as a delivery system for bitter herbs, at least until a person's palate adjusts to the taste of bitter. Digestive bitters must actually be tasted in order to work. Without that bitter taste to signal salivation to start, a digestive bitter just doesn't work on the liver, although the herb's other properties may still work. The sour, pungent, and spicy flavors of fire cider do not mask the bitter taste, but it makes the bitter taste far easier to tolerate.

CHRONIC MALNUTRITION = CHRONIC ILLNESS

I'm convinced that our lack of proper nutrition is at the heart of the chronic illness epidemic in the United States. According to data from the Centers for Disease Control and Prevention (CDC) website:

+ 1 in every 2 Americans has a chronic disease.

+ 75% of medical expenses are due to chronic disease.

+ 70% of all deaths are attributable to chronic disease.

Those three statistics are enough to tell you that something is dreadfully wrong with our standard approach to health. This is in every way an indictment of our highly politicized health care system, which is more rightly called a "sick care system," and our industrialized food system. Maintenance drugs are gold mines for pharmaceutical companies, which provide a way to stay well enough not to complain, but not well enough to feel truly healthy.

Judging by the CDC's statistics, most of us are in some way sick. We have been sick for so long that I don't think many people really know what "well" feels like anymore. "Well" is something we may vaguely remember from childhood, before aches and pains, excess weight, and high blood pressure set in.

What we can do is to begin intensely feeding our cells with nutrient-dense herbs and seaweeds, reduce sugars, replace table salt with unadulterated sea salt, and add plenty of lacto-fermented foods, such as homemade yogurt, sauerkraut, kimchi, and beet kvass. We can begin to loosen our joints and force the tissues to use the glucose in blood for energy with a simple walk, perhaps in an aromatic evergreen forest, where the essential oils we sniff from pines can help support our immune function. And where our bodies require a little extra help, we can work with herbs to support the body's natural healing processes. This sounds like an actual "health care plan" to me.

If you have a chronic illness, it is imperative to do what you can to improve your health. Any effort is well worthwhile. Chronic illness raises your risks of catching an infectious disease and suffering a serious complication from that infectious disease, and it slows recovery time and keeps wounds from healing. As the outbreak of MERS coronavirus in Saudi Arabia demonstrated quite clearly, chronic illness is a major risk. When the MERS outbreak began in 2012, it had a fatality rate of 60%. Of those who died, 96% had underlying, chronic illnesses. Topping the list was diabetes at 68%, followed by chronic renal disease (49%), hypertension (34%), and chronic cardiac disease (28%).[18]

Some of the most common chronic illnesses in the United States are obesity, hypertension, diabetes, and arthritis. Let's take a look at each of these individually.

---

18   Abdullah Assiri et al.,"Epidemiological, Demographic, and Clinical Characteristics of 47 Cases of Middle East Respiratory Syndrome Coronavirus Disease from Saudi Arabia: A Descriptive Study," *The Lancet Infectious Diseases* 13, no. 9 (2013): 752–61.

OBESITY

Reducing body fat lowers the risks of developing a number of chronic illnesses. Obesity is defined as having a body mass index (BMI) of 30% or more. It is linked to metabolic syndrome, which is also associated with cardiovascular disease, cancer, diabetes, hypertension, high cholesterol, and PCOS. If you are obese, you will ultimately put more stress and strain on your joints, aggravating any arthritis that may develop.

The causes of obesity are many. While overeating and lack of movement are the main causes, they are not the only causes. Has there been an overuse of antibiotics that changed the bacteria in the gut, allowing candida to thrive? Candida can drive a person to eat more sugar. Its not a question of willpower, it's a compulsion. One of the bifidobacteria, part of the healthy bacteria populations which antibiotics can kill, has been shown to cause the body to use calories at a faster rate. Berberine can be a massive help as it holds candida at bay while not harming the beneficial helpful bacteria in the gut. This allows the gut flora to return to a healthy balance. Berberine can play a pivotal role in combatting insulin resistance, a well-known risk factor for obesity. If you need some help fighting the battle of the bulge, try any of the berberine herbs taken in tincture form, 30 to 60 drops, 3 times per day, 30 minutes before each meal.

Lack of movement seems built into our days. Hours at a desk, working at a computer, and relaxation at home on a couch watching television do not add up to post-disaster, survival fitness. If you identify with the couch potato I just described, I encourage you to reconsider how you spend your relaxation time. Could you walk to your bug out location? Could you haul water if you had to? Could you carry a spouse or a child who was injured to a safe place? Maybe an easy hike this weekend is in order to get the blood pumping again.

I suggest eliminating excess sugar; adding some healthy fats like coconut oil, avocado, and cold water fish; eating more whole foods and less processed foods; moving more; drinking more water; and getting more rest. If that doesn't encourage the body to release excess weight, then I suggest a hybrid of Nutritional Syrup and Traditional Fire Cider. This will cut way down on any sugar from the syrup, and should load the body with missing nutrients. The ingredients are mostly available in dried form, but use fresh whenever possible.

✿ CAT'S FITNESS TONIC ✿

5 parts nettle leaves

5 parts hibiscus flowers

4 parts horsetail

4 parts ginger root (as fresh as possible)

3 parts turmeric root (if fresh, otherwise 3 heaping tablespoons, dried)

3 parts cayenne (as red pepper flakes)

2 parts parsley

2 parts rose hips

2 parts *Gymnema sylvestre* (only available for sale as dried herb in the U.S.)

2 parts Siberian ginseng

1 part onion

1 part garlic

1 part horseradish

Apple cider vinegar

Lemon juice

Yacon syrup

Dandelion tincture

Burdock tincture

Coptis tincture

1 Using protective gloves (for the red pepper flakes), mix all herbs (nettles leaves through horseradish) thoroughly in a really big bowl.

2 Because of the fresh ginger root, you won't be able to store this remedy. Instead, get as many quart mason jars as you need, or a pickle jar, to contain all the herbs. Cover with apple cider vinegar. Allow to steep for 2 to 4 weeks.

3 Strain the herbs, and measure the volume of herbal vinegar recovered. Add one-quarter the volume of the apple cider vinegar in lemon juice, and one-quarter the volume of the apple cider vinegar in yacon syrup.

This is fine to take as is, but adding bitter herbs (dandelion and burdock) will help the liver, especially in anyone suffering from fatty liver disease. The addition of coptis helps to keep candida and the "bad" bacteria at bay while not harming any of the beneficial bacteria. This will give the beneficial bacteria a chance to recolonize the colon.

Take 2 ounces of this remedy in 2 ounces of apple juice, and add 60 drops of the blended tincture.

Take 3 times daily, 30 minutes before each meal, for 6 weeks, then evaluate how this remedy impacted your other weight-loss efforts.

It can take at least 6 weeks for a body that has been negatively impacted by fluctuating insulin levels for years to show weight loss. A relatively healthy person can lose weight in a short period of time, but a hormonal component may come into play, making weight loss more difficult.

SEAWEED, SALT, AND HYPERTENSION

A natural source of minerals, seaweeds provide excellent nutrition. They are nutrient dense and mineral rich, and contain natural iodine. Just like natural, unadulterated sea salt (which is gray or light pink, unlike white salt, which is refined and had its minerals stripped), sea vegetables work with natural iodine to keep our bodies healthy.

A public relations war against sodium has been raging for years. The FDA, the medical industry, and various associations (American Heart Association, American Stroke Association, and the rest) have all been banging on about sodium, and promoting low-sodium foods as healthy.

As is all too common, the science fails to translate into the political arena of health policy. There is no evidence that unadulterated salt with all of its minerals intact raises blood pressure. Research going all the way back to the 1980s shows no clear link between eating a low-sodium diet and lowering blood pressure.[19, 20] Even worse, evidence shows that a low-sodium diet not only fails to lower elevated blood pressure, but it is associated with higher mortality,[21] worse outcomes for individuals with congestive heart failure

---

19   "Intersalt: An International Study of Electrolyte Excretion and Blood Pressure. Results for 24 Hour Urinary Sodium and Potassium Excretion. Intersalt Cooperative Research Group," *British Medical Journal* 297 (1988): 319–28.

20   Judy Z. Miller et al., "Heterogeneity of Blood Pressure Response to Dietary Sodium Restriction in Normotensive Adults," *Journal of Chronic Diseases* 40, no. 3 (1986): 245–50.

21   H. Cohen et al., "Sodium Intake and Mortality in the NHANES II Follow-up Study," the *American Journal of Medicine* 119, no. 3 (2006): 275.e7–75.e14.

because of detrimental effects on the kidneys,[22] increased risk of fractures in the elderly not associated with falls,[23] and a higher risk of death from heart disease.[24]

This is not to suggest that consuming large amounts of table salt is healthy. The takeaway is that lowering sodium intake does not provide the benefits we have been led to believe. There is surely too much sodium in processed foods. There is little difference between the salt used in commercially prepared foods and table salt, other than that table salt has added iodine, although a surprisingly low amount of it. What we are left with is a nutritionally bereft, processed white salt, lacking any of the minerals that would actually help maintain healthy blood pressure levels, with a tiny amount of iodine added in.

Iodine can be a help or a harm. Some people are allergic to iodine and should not consume it. If you consumed too much iodine on a regular basis, you could develop hyperthyroidism (overactive thyroid gland). If you ever tasted the full flavor of seaweeds and true sea salt, however, you know the intense flavors make it unlikely that you would overeat these foods.

If you happen to live close to the shore, you're in luck as you can harvest your own seaweed. If not, you can order dried seaweed in larger amounts and stock them in your pantry. They can be used like salt, to flavor soups and sauces, and to add to seasoning blends. If you do not like the oceanic taste of seaweed , then you can powder and encapsulate them. A single size 0 capsule daily should suffice.

22 Salvatore Paterna et al., "Normal-Sodium Diet Compared with Low-Sodium Diet in Compensated Congestive Heart Failure: Is Sodium an Old Enemy or a New Friend?" *Clinical Science* 114, no. 3 (2008): 221–30.

23 Ewout J. Hoorn et al., "Mild Hyponatremia as a Risk Factor for Fractures: The Rotterdam Study," *Journal of Bone and Mineral Research* 26, no. 8 (2011): 1822–828.

24 K. Stolarz-Skrzypek et al., "Fatal and Nonfatal Outcomes, Incidence of Hypertension, and Blood Pressure Changes in Relation to Urinary Sodium Excretion," *JAMA: The Journal of the American Medical Association* 305, no. 17 (2011): 1777–785.

HYPERTENSION

Hypertension is nothing to mess around with. You can have it and not know it. There may not be any warning signs unless you actively check your blood pressure—a great reason to have a blood pressure cuff, and to include some type of routine health evaluation as part of your preps. Resist the urge to take, retake, and retake your blood pressure. Taking a reading from the same arm twice in a row can create an artificially high reading.

My concern for people with hypertension during a disaster is that the only measure of control they have over their blood pressure is a pill. Pharmacies will be one of the very first places to be raided after a crisis. Most instances of hypertension are directly related to lifestyle (diet, exercise, smoking). It is well worth the effort to take control of your blood pressure now while times are still good.

Hypertension is not normal. It's not a part of normal aging. Something is causing it. Is it diet? Stress? A kidney problem? It's impossible for me to give a single remedy for hypertension because there are many causes. However, if you switch your source of carbohydrates from breads and grains to vegetables, feed your cells with deep nutrition, and ditch the table salt in favor of sea salt, you may find that your body begins to correct itself. Many of Traditional Fire Cider's ingredients make the tonic a good choice but a few additions will improve the remedy for hypertension.

❦ HEART HELPER TONIC ❦

Garlic

Ginger root

Cayenne

Nettle seeds

Red sage (Salvia miltiorrhiza)

Hawthorn berries

Celery seed (Apium graveolens, v. dulce)

Turmeric

Horseradish

Onion

Apple cider vinegar

Lemon juice

Honey

1   Layer the ingredients in a quart or larger mason jar as desired, and cover with apple cider vinegar.

2   Allow to steep for 2 to 4 weeks

3   Strain the herbs, and reserve the liquid.

4   To the liquid, add lemon juice and honey to taste.

Take 1 ounce straight or diluted in apple juice 2 or 3 times daily.

None of these herbs will artificially lower blood pressure. If you have normal blood pressure, it won't drop if you take this remedy. These ingredients only encourage cardiovascular health. Be sure to check your blood pressure regularly, preferably at the same time every day.

You may also wish to speak to your doctor about different blood pressure–lowering prescriptions. Certain prescriptions can be stopped cold turkey (not advisable), as will happen if we suddenly find ourselves in TEOTWAWKI. Others cannot, and stopping them suddenly poses a significant risk.

DIABETES

One thing I often encounter in preparedness forums is the assertion that nothing can be done for type 1 diabetics post-disaster. Yes, type 2 diabetes can be addressed through diet and herbs, but that doesn't mean that nothing can be done for type 1 diabetics.

I have not had the opportunity to work with many type 1 diabetics. My sample size is limited to what I can count on one hand. However, what I have been fortunate to observe mirrors what was shown through a study done in India on *Gymnema sylvestre*. In India's traditional healing system, Ayurveda, gymnema is known as the "destroyer of sugar." It has been used to reverse both type 1 and type 2 diabetes, and there is a growing body of literature to support this, easily searchable on PubMed.gov.

I have observed the use of gymnema leaves extracted with grain alcohol and also with vinegar. The alcohol extraction seems to work better, but the vinegar extraction is more pleasing to the palate. What I have observed in those who continued with the remedy, using either extraction, is that the need for insulin lessened, but the change was exceptionally gradual. And in our world of fast food and quick fixes, some people stop taking it because it simply doesn't work fast enough.

The study in India resulted in 60% of people being able to completely reverse their type 1 diabetes after 18 months. The remaining 40% were able to reduce their amount of insulin, and some came off insulin completely. However, they had to remain on gymnema. Unfortunately, there is no way to know if they would be able to come off gymnema if given more time.

It's true. Gymnema takes a long time to work, and may not work for everyone. However, it has been shown to regenerate the beta cells in the pancreas to allow a person to start making insulin. It also seems to help the body use the insulin more efficiently.[25] It has been used with even greater success in type 2 diabetes and in addressing obesity. Unfortunately, only the dried herb and not the plant itself is available in the United States.

Fenugreek is another herb that has shown a similar but an even slower action in regenerating the beta cells of the pancreas. However, it is easy to get fenugreek seeds here. Berberine can also be a significant help in diabetes care. As documented in Kerry Bone's book, *Practices and Principals of Phytotherapy*, berberine was shown to work as well as metformin at controlling post-meal rises in blood sugar. Plus a study done in China showed that berberine can prevent pancreatic beta cell apoptosis,[26] which may preventing the disease from worsening.

ARTHRITIS

Arthritis is a very painful irritation of the joints. The two most common types are osteoarthritis and rheumatoid arthritis, the latter being an autoimmune disease. The most immediately effective remedy I've found is Pain Relief Salve (page 146) containing cayenne. Other arthritis remedies include:

Nettle tea. Nettle relieves swelling around joints and moves excess fluids. I've found it useful in reducing symptoms in autoimmune diseases.

---

25   E. R. Shanmugasundaram et al., "Use of Gymnema Sylvestre Leaf Extract in the Control of Blood Glucose in Insulin-Dependent Diabetes Mellitus," *Journal of Ethnopharmacology* 30, no. 3 (1990): 281–94.

26   S. Wu et al., "Effects of Berberine on the Pancreatic Beta Cell Apoptosis in Rats with Insulin Resistance," *Zhongguo Zhong Xi Yi Jie He Za Zhi* 31 (October 2011): 1383–38.

White willow tea. The bark (see page 116) has a similar effect on pain as aspirin.

Cayenne. Use topically or ingest to lower inflammation because cayenne contains capsaicin in abundance. If too strong a flavor, take via capsules.

Arnica. This effective pain relief herb can easily be made into a salve.

Comfrey. It works well to relieve pain, especially when combined with arnica.

Birch bark tea. Birch bark works similarly to white willow bark.

Ginger-turmeric milk. Gently simmer two pieces of ginger root, each the size of your thumb, in a pot with 4 cups of any milk you wish (dairy, almond, coconut) for 10 minutes. Make sure not to let it bubble over. Add 1 heaping teaspoon of turmeric, and allow to steep for 20 minutes. Strain using a fine-mesh strainer, cheesecloth, or muslin—or use a French press, as I do. Add honey to taste, and drink throughout the day.

ASTHMA

For some, asthma is a lifelong condition that can occasionally be improved, but it's never going to go away. For others, it comes on later in life and may be related to food allergies. Eliminating the allergen should solve the problem. In either case, herbs may be able to help reduce the effects of asthma. Two of the herbs used for acute attacks are lobelia and ma huang, also known as ephedra. Each of these herbs comes with cautions about its use.

Lobelia was widely used by Native Americans and has a long history of safe use. However, this highly effective antispasmodic herb is given only as a low-dose tincture and is not for people with a weak or compromised heart. See page 93 for more information on lobelia.

Ephedra was taken off the market, not for being unsafe, but because it was misused. It was exploited as a weight-loss supplement in doses that would not occur in nature, and people took more than the recommended dosage of that already unnaturally high dose.

While the sale of ephedra was banned, growing it is still legal. Check out the Resource section for seeds (page 220). Ephedra can elevate blood pressure, so take it slow in getting to know this herb. Related plants that are somewhat less potent, such as Mormon tea, can be used instead.

Keep in mind that every person is different. Not every remedy works for everyone. This is true even of pharmaceuticals. If it were me and I were concerned about asthma, I wouldn't wait until a crisis to see what works for me and what doesn't. I would try the herbs now, while life is relatively calm. I also recommend working with a skilled herbalist. Always use common sense and keep your safety in mind when getting to know asthma herbs.

ACUTE REMEDIES

Hot coffee. Hot coffee taken at the start of an asthma attack can sometimes stop the bout from developing into a full-blown attack. (I also find coffee useful with bronchitis.) Both the caffeine and the heat have a beneficial effect.

Hot herbal tea. Hot herbal tea made from 2 parts elecampagne, 2 parts mullein, and 1 part ma huang.

Steam inhalation. A steam inhalation of rosemary, thyme, and sage. Be safe: Remove the mixture from the heat source, as steam can burn.

Cramp bark tincture. Take 30 drops either under the tongue (faster effect) or diluted in water or juice, taken every 30 minutes until the attack subsides.

Lobelia tincture. Use 2 parts lobelia tincture combined with 1 part cayenne tincture, 20 drops taken every 30 minutes. Do not exceed 4 doses at the 30-minute intervals. If this does not work, you will have to move on to another remedy. It is not recommended to take too much lobelia.

PREVENTION/REDUCTION OF ATTACKS

Tincture blend of 3 parts *Grindelia robusta,* 2 parts mullein, and 1 part dong quai *(Angelica sinensis)* taken in water or added to Herbal Tussin Tea (page 150). Start with 30 drops once daily. Slowly increase either the dose or frequency (but not both at the same time) until you notice a difference.

SEASONAL ALLERGIES

As miserable as a bad cold is, seasonal allergies are worse. They come at the most inconvenient times. Imagine trying to plant your vegetable garden in the spring—or harvest your garden, pick apples, or prep the garden beds for a winter crop—while dealing with allergies. For some, allergies are mild, annoying symptoms. For others, allergy season is pure misery.

For allergies, I suggest a two-fold approach: First, treat the liver and, second, take an anti-allergy tea blend. The liver produces antihistamines and needs plenty of support when you are experiencing allergies. Add digestive bitter herbs to your allergy plan—such as dandelion, burdock, milk thistle, gentian, wood betony, and berberine—to support proper liver function.

The anti-allergy tea includes butterbur, which contains pyrrolizidine alkaloids (PA), just as comfrey does. But for occasional use, such as seasonal allergies, which tend to last for a week or two at a time, I wouldn't worry about the alkaloids. Butterbur has a long history of treating both allergy and asthma symptoms. However, anyone with liver disease should avoid using butterbur.

The tea also includes nettle leaves, another source of antihistamines, which are a great help for seasonal allergies as well as for tamping down many inflammatory responses. The surprise to many is the inclusion of goldenrod. Goldenrod does not cause hayfever, and it isn't even related to the plant that does. Instead, it is a powerful remedy against hayfever and other seasonal allergies.

To make the tea, combine the following herbs in the proportions below. If you are uncomfortable with including butterbur, just leave it out. If you will be using this tea for other allergies on an ongoing basis, like pet or dust allergies, definitely leave out the butterbur.

❧ ANTI-ALLERGY TEA ❧

4 parts nettle leaves   **3 parts goldenrod**   **1 part eyebright**

3 parts butterbur   **2 parts peppermint**

1   Blend the dried herbs in a large batch to have on hand when needed.

2   To brew a cup of the tea, steep 1 teaspoon of the mixed, dried herbs in 6 to 8 ounces of hot water. Allow to steep, covered, for at least 15 minutes.

3   Sweeten with honey, and drink as needed for allergy relief.

For severe allergic reactions, such an anaphylaxis, see page 123.

COMMON COLD/FLU

Sometimes it is impossible to tell a cold from the flu at the onset. My strategy is to combine both elderberry and two herbs that are effective against rhinovirus, echinacea and ginger. This way, no matter if it is a cold or a flu, treatment can start immediately. The following elixir can be a big help during cold and flu season. However, for the echinacea to work, it has to be taken immediately when symptoms begin, and taken frequently. I have sometimes swapped out the echinacea for rose hips. You could make this into a syrup for the kids, but I want to give at least one recipe as an elixir—so keep this remedy for the adults.

❦ ELDERBERRY AND ❦ ECHINACEA ELIXIR

½ cup dried elderberries

½ cup *Echinacea angustifolia* root

½ cup ginger root, peeled and chopped

Approximately 2 cups brandy

3 to 6 lemon slices

4 to 5 cinnamon sticks

Approximately 2 cups raw honey

1 Place the elderberries, echinacea, and ginger in a pint mason jar.

2 Fill the jar to the top with your favorite brandy, and allow to steep for 4 to 6 weeks.

3 Put the lemon and cinnamon in another pint jar, and fill the jar with honey. Allow to steep for 4 to 6 weeks.

4 Strain the herbs from both the brandy and the honey.

5 Combine the strained brandy and honey. Bottle the mixture, and label it.

6 Take 1 teaspoon every hour for the first day. Stay at home and relax. From the second day on, back down to 1 teaspoon every 3 to 4 hours.

❦ NATURAL FLU SYRUP ❦

Nothing is more effective for the flu than elderberry syrup, another of my staple remedies. Star anise comes in a close second, but more people will have access to elderberry bushes than star anise in a post-disaster situation. The blogosphere is loaded with recipes for elderberry syrup these days. I've been making this remedy for years and have developed many versions of it. It makes a tasty syrup that even kids enjoy taking. You can use the syrup to make homemade gummy candies and as a topping for homemade yogurt.

½ cup dried elderberries

1 piece of ginger (the size of your thumb), peeled and sliced

4 to 5 garlic cloves

⅛ cup cinnamon bark chips

9 whole cloves

2 cups water

1½ cups honey

1 Make a double decoction of the elderberries, ginger, garlic, cinnamon chips, and cloves.

2 Strain the herbs, squeezing out all the liquid you can.

3 While the liquid is still warm, add honey to equal 16 ounces (2 cups).

Take every hour at the onset of symptoms, and then every 3 to 4 hours the next day. Continue taking as needed until symptoms are gone, or just because you like the taste.

DIAPER RASH

My son never had a single case of diaper rash. My daughter, however, seemed prone to rashes. Thankfully, they never got out of hand, and I credit calendula for that. First, infuse calendula flowers in coconut oil (both of these substances are fungus-fighting skin healers). I would do this in a slow cooker on warm for 2 full weeks (shutting down the slow cooker at night) because I prefer a good, strong infusion for my infused oils, although a weak, but usable, oil would be ready in 2 hours. Rather than just calendula flowers, you could also use a 50/50 blend of calendula and chamomile flowers. And instead of using only coconut oil, you could use combination of coconut and rose hip seed oil, which is a bit pricey but an excellent skin healer. Diaper rash can easily lead to broken skin, and rose hip seed oil is very helpful in wound healing.

Also in this recipe is mango butter and a powder, either corn starch or arrowroot powder. The blending of the solid fat of the mango butter (which has a higher melting point than the coconut oil) with the liquid oils produces a more solid, buttery product which is spreadable, not dripping. The powder reduces the oily feeling. I included mango butter because that is what I used to make this when my daughter was in diapers. If you did not have access to mango butter post-disaster, substitute lard or tallow. These are probably in your storage pantry anyway, along with the corn starch.

❦ ANTIFUNGAL BABY BALM ❦

4 ounces calendula infused coconut oil

1 ounce rose hip seed oil (or another ounce of calendula infused coconut oil, if you don't have rose hip seed oil

3 ounces mango butter

1 teaspoon corn starch or arrowroot powder (more if needed)

1   Gently melt the oils and the butter in a double boiler.

2   Once they have completely melted and incorporated, remove from the heat.

3   As the oils begin to cool, the balm will start to solidify. Add either corn starch or arrowroot powder.

4   Using an immersion blender, incorporate the powder into the balm. If the balm seems too greasy or feels too loose, add another teaspoon of powder. Fully incorporate the powder into the balm.

5   Scoop the balm into a container and label it. Make sure hands are clean when touching the balm.

6   Gently clean baby's bottom. Apply a thick coat to the rash, and expect some to end up soaking into the diaper.

7   Change diapers frequently.

Don't discount the value of just letting a baby have some diaper-free time. Getting air to a rash can do wonders to clear it quickly.

If you wanted a remedy to treat or prevent fungal skin infections in adults, especially on feet, you could adjust this formula by adding peppermint and tea tree oils (in 1% of total volume each) to the basic formula. This will add to the antifungal properties of the balm, as well as bring cooling relief to itchy feet.

NAUSEA AND INTESTINAL INFECTIONS

Ginger infused honey might sound like a tasty treat. And it really is. In fact, you could use it to make a glaze for chicken, but that's not why I've included it here. Ginger is excellent for nausea and calms the intense intestinal cramping associated with various intestinal infections. With the addition of a few more ingredients, this syrup is warming, tasty, sweet, and intended to make the sick person more comfortable.

🐝 GINGER-INFUSED HONEY 🐝

2 pieces of ginger (each the size of your thumbs)

½ lemon, sliced

¼ cup cinnamon bark chips

¼ cup chamomile flowers

15 whole cloves

10 cardamom pods

Approximately 2 cups honey

1   Fill a pint mason jar with the ginger, lemon, cinnamon chips, chamomile, cloves, and cardamom.

2   Cover with honey, and fill to equal 16 ounces (2 cups).

3   Allow to steep for 6 weeks.

4   To strain, gently warm the jar by placing it in an inch or two of water in a slow cooker set to warm. Warming the honey makes it runny and easier to strain.

5   Strain the herbs, and bottle the honey.

6   Take by the teaspoon as needed.

CHRONIC INTESTINAL DISCOMFORTS

Your choice of an anti-diarrhea remedy will depend on what's causing the diarrhea. A flare-up of colitis and a salmonella infection aren't handled in the same way. Ulcerative colitis, Crohn's disease, and irritable bowel syndrome are miserable and absolutely need an effective remedy.

In general, oak bark tea can help stop the symptoms, but peppermint tea can also be a big help in calming the cramps. Peppermint is also much gentler (and better tasting) for children. Ginger helps to calm cramping too, while ginger's cousin turmeric helps reduce inflammation. Ginger is most effective when juiced, but the taste is quite intense. Making a decoction flavored with honey and lemon is often more palatable. If you want the juice, you could add another juice, such as carrot or apple, to dilute the heat somewhat.

Ultimately, the remedy for these chronic intestinal conditions lies in healing the gut. It isn't a quick fix, but a long-term commitment. The best way I have found for healing the gut is the GAPS protocol. GAPS stands for both Gut and Psychology Syndrome, as well as Gut and Physiology Syndrome. Both titles refer to the same protocol. The idea behind GAPS is to remove any potential irritant to the intestine from the diet, supplement with fermented foods and probiotics, and soothe the gut with plenty of bone broth. All grains are eliminated, and then slowly brought back over time, to see if they can be tolerated. This provides the gut with an opportunity to heal.

The nice thing about fermented foods, besides the fact that they are loaded with beneficial bacteria, is that lacto-fermentation extends the shelf life of your produce. If you keep these items in a cool location away from sunlight, you should be able to consume fresh, lacto-fermented foods throughout winter. Of course, you can make them throughout summer as well, but having fresh food in winter without importing it is quite special. And by fermenting food, not only are you getting an inexpensive probiotic supplement, but the nutrients are made more bioavailable.

WOMEN'S NATURAL MEDICINE

Women have unique health concerns that have to be taken into consideration when preparing for long-term emergencies. Thankfully, natural remedies can help relieve many of the common complaints women experience throughout the various stages of life. This section covers common complaints in each phase of a woman's life, as well as remedies to assist pregnancy and options for birth control. Because of the specialized nature of this section, I have included more herbs than I did in Chapter 4, Materia Medica.

For a better understanding of birth and complications, as well as how to support a woman through this process and how to assess the health of a newborn, see the books listed in Resources (page 216).

PREMENSTRUAL SYNDROME (PMS)

PMS is often marked by mood swings, crying, anger, depression, abdominal cramping, and swelling. It is not restricted to just the week prior to menstruation. For many, PMS symptoms may begin a week or so before menstruation starts but almost always continues into the cycle itself.

Stress, poor nutrition, and lack of sanitary conditions are some of the common concerns to expect post-collapse. These situations can cause or exacerbate delayed menstruation, acne, urinary tract infections, and yeast infections.

Pay attention to the quality of your food storage. When good nutrition, such as plenty of B6, B12, and healthy fats, are not enough to keep PMS at bay, consider the following herbs:

Nettle leaves. Take this nutritive, mild diuretic as a tea to help with excess water weight.

Dandelion leaves. Use this diuretic in a salad or cook it as you would spinach.

Ginger root. Use fresh in a decoction to relieve smooth muscle tissue from spasms.

Cramp bark. Take as a tincture to relieve cramps.

Motherwort. Take as a tincture to relieve moodiness.

Black cohosh. Take as a tincture to encourage ovulation and for its antispasmodic properties, which alleviate cramping.

Codonopsis. Take as a tincture in case of a hormone-triggered migraine.

Finally, a comfort measure worth mentioning for menstrual cramping is to hold a hot water bottle to the abdomen.

BIRTH CONTROL

Birth control during and after a major disaster is problematic. Options from the mainstream medical world include long-term hormonal birth control implanted into the arm, an inserted IUD, or a stockpile of months' worth of consumables (birth control pills, spermicidal films, spermicidal foams, and condoms).

Each has positive and negative points. Hormonal-based birth control is effective, but for many women it only exacerbates underlying hormone imbalances. Hormone-based birth control can also raise the risk or serious side effects, such as heart attack, stroke, and cancer. Implanted devices, hormonal or otherwise, at some point must be removed. In an uncertain future, I am not positive that is the wisest choice. I have a friend whose IUD has perforated her uterus twice. Personally, I wouldn't risk that in a post-collapse situation.

Another drawback of hormone-based contraception is that it offers no protection against sexually transmitted diseases. Only condoms offer that, and they are not 100% reliable. This is a worrisome thought as gonorrhea increasingly becomes more antibiotic resistant.

Birth control, no matter your opinion of it, serves a vital function after a disaster. When your circumstances are dire, and you are having trouble keeping yourself alive, it's probably not the opportune time to get pregnant. This may be especially true if you previously had a birth with complications. While pregnancy and labor are not illnesses, and both are normal processes, a disaster is not a normal circumstance.

Two options for natural birth control are the Fertility Awareness Method (FAM) and wild carrot seeds *(Daucus carota)*. First, let me state that

FAM is not the rhythm method. Yes, it involves charts, but it is far more accurate, and well worth your time and effort.

FAM uses consistent, ongoing observation of three key ovulation indicators: basal body temperature, cervical fluids, and cervical position. It is a dynamic assessment of what is going on in your body at any given time, as opposed to merely an estimate of what might be going on in your body, and far more accurate then subtracting 2 weeks as is done in the rhythm method.

Beyond just knowing when you are fertile to avoid pregnancy, or perhaps in order to become pregnant, understanding your cycle is understanding your body. Having a period is not evidence of ovulation. By using the FAM method, you can determine if ovulation is even happening. This is very important in understanding your reproductive health and being alert to a potential hormonal imbalance, fertility issue, or menopause. For more information on FAM, see *Taking Charge of Your Fertility* by Toni Weschler.

Herbalist Robin Rose Bennett has done some small-scale studies on the use of wild carrot seeds as birth control. She has posted much of her findings on her website, RobinRoseBennett.com, and I strongly encourage any woman who is looking for a natural birth control option to read all of the information she has put together on the subject.

According to Robin, wild carrot seeds have an extremely long history in birth control, as far back as the 4th or 5th century BCE. Hippocrates compiled the first written record. Wild carrot seeds also have a long history right here in the United States. In Appalachia, the seeds have been used for generations to prevent pregnancy by preventing implantation.

Over the years, Robin has adjusted her recommendations. Currently, she recommends making a tincture of the wild carrot seeds and flowers. The resulting tincture should smell strongly of carrots. Taking the tincture daily may actually weaken the effect. The best results occur when the tincture is taken within 8 hours after intercourse. Take a dose of 30 to 60 drops, 3 times daily, every 8 hours.

Caution: Wild carrot, also known as Queen Anne's lace, looks similar to another plant, poison hemlock. However, plant identification should be fairly straightforward. A very easy way to tell the two plants apart is by the stem. Queen Anne's lace has hairy stems, and wild carrot does not. One of my herbal teachers, Linda Patterson, told our class to remember "The queen has hairy legs."

PREGNANCY

Although the timing may not be opportune, doubtless there will still be pregnancies and births post-disaster. It is your job to help make a woman more comfortable during pregnancy with some herbal remedies, when and if she needs them. Again, this section deals only with normal birth. Please seek out the midwifery books in Resources (page 217) to get an idea of all the variations of "normal birth" and how to handle the unexpected during a pregnancy or labor.

As important as nutrition is during pregnancy, it is also important prior to pregnancy. In fact, the benefits from folate are largely based on the folate stores prior to conception. If you believe that there a chance you could become pregnant, start taking Nutritional Syrup (page 166) or try this simple, nourishing tea. Note that the measurements of herbs is by weight.

❦ HEALTHY MOMMA TEA ❦

½ ounce red raspberry leaves   ¼ ounce nettle leaves   ¼ ounce milky oat tops or oatstraw

1   Put all herbs into a quart mason jar, and pour boiling water over them.

2   Allow to steep for 2 hours, strain, and take up to 4 cups daily.

Red raspberry leaf is an important herb for women, especially pregnant women. Some people, however, mistakenly think that it can induce labor. It does not cause the onset of labor. However, it can increase Braxton Hicks contractions, or as I prefer to call them, "practice contractions," if a woman starts taking red raspberry leaf late in pregnancy. If she has been taking it since the beginning of the pregnancy, there are no noticeable differences in the intensity or frequency of the practice contractions.

Nausea is one of the most common complaints during the first trimester. It can be caused by the surge of estrogen at this time, but nausea or morning sickness can happen at any time of the day, during any trimester, because of excess estrogen, low vitamin B6 levels, and low blood sugar.

Try more protein-based snacks, as long as there is no allergy to nuts, sunflower seeds, pumpkin seeds, and cheese. Munching these snacks first thing in the morning can help mitigate low blood sugar and the need for extra B6.

Ginger is a time-tested remedy for nausea. Candied ginger is a very convenient way to carry and consume ginger on the go. Ginger and peppermint tea with lemon, or either ginger or peppermint on its own, does a good job of calming morning sickness.

Always try to stay hydrated, as dehydration can cause nausea. Dandelion and yellow dock added to the Nutritional Syrup can help the liver process the excess estrogen that causes nausea in early pregnancy.

Anemia is a common problem during pregnancy. If you notice signs of anemia, such as fatigue, weakness, dizziness, paleness, shortness of breath, chest pain, or headaches, it might be time for Yellow Dock and Molasses Syrup, a common remedy to supplement iron levels. But unlike most iron supplements, it doesn't cause constipation. In fact, yellow dock is a gentle, self-regulating laxative. Considering how pregnancy can constipate a woman, this is a welcome change. Yellow dock is a wonderful digestive herb providing not only iron, but relief from indigestion, gas, and jaundice.

To make the syrup, follow these direction or simply just add yellow dock to the Nutritional Syrup recipe. Note that the measurement of yellow dock is by weight, and the measurement of liquids by volume.

❧ YELLOW DOCK AND ❧ MOLASSES SYRUP

1 ounce yellow dock root	1 quart water	⅔ cup molasses

1   Make a decoction of the yellow dock and the water.

2   Strain the herbs, reserving the liquid.

3   Add the molasses to the strained liquid, and stir to incorporate.

4   Store in the refrigerator for up to 6 months.

5   Take ½ to 1 teaspoon 2 times per day.

MISCARRIAGE

Miscarriage is a difficult subject, but considering that approximately 10% to 20% of pregnancies result in miscarriage, it is important to be prepared for such an event. Miscarriage is a loss of a pregnancy prior to 20 weeks. Often, there is nothing that can be done to prevent a miscarriage. There was something wrong: The fetus was not viable, and the mother's body recognized this fact and rejected the fetus. Occasionally, however, miscarriage can be linked to chemicals in the environment or an underlying hormonal imbalance.

If you suspect the possibility of miscarriage or loss of the pregnancy during any trimester, proceed as follows:

+ Get plenty of bed rest.

+ Increase fluids.

+ Increase protein intake.

+ Supplement with 2,000 IUs of vitamin E, once daily.

+ Supplement with 500 mg of vitamin C, once daily.

+ Avoid intercourse.

+ Wait to see if uterine contractions slow down or cease.

Dehydration is a very common trigger for miscarriage. Vitamins E and C are known for helping to encourage fetal attachment to the uterine wall. While there is no solid evidence that bed rest is effective at preventing miscarriage, movement is known to encourage labor. So I would play it safe, and limit movement.

If contractions do not slow down or cease, choose ONE of the following:

+ Cramp bark decoction, 2 to 5 times per day.

+ Lobelia tincture, 1 to 5 drops in 8 ounces of water, every 30 to 60 minutes until cramping slows down.

How you prepare cramp bark determines the kind of effect it has. When taken as a tincture, it makes contractions more productive. This is perfect for cramps associated with menstruation, but less so for preventing miscarriage. For a miscarriage, a decoction brings out cramp bark's antispasmodic properties instead.

Lobelia is the supreme antispasmodic. However, this also makes it a low-dose herb. Hopefully, relaxing the uterus will stop the miscarriage. Unfortunately, neither herbs nor pharmaceuticals can make any guarantee about preventing a miscarriage.

POSTPARTUM CARE

Assuming a normal, healthy birth has occurred, stay around to help clean up, as mom will have enough to do. When mom is ready, breastfeeding with skin to skin contact helps the bonding process, and it also helps mom's uterus properly expel the placenta. Further nursing helps prevent postpartum hemorrhage.

If mom wants it, motherwort is a helpful herb at this point. It helps the uterus contract and the placenta separate from the uterus. Motherwort helps with afterpains, preventing postpartum hemorrhage and establishing the milk supply. Goat's rue *(Galega officinalis)* is another herb that can increase the milk supply.

Although not popular in our culture, eating the placenta is a part of traditional Chinese medicine. While not everyone wants to dine on a placenta sandwich, the placenta can be dehydrated and encapsulated. This is supposed to increase milk production and lower the risks of postpartum depression as well as uterine hemorrhage.

In case of uterine hemorrhage, shepherd's purse *(Capsella bursa-pastoris)* or yarrow tincture is a good option. I prefer shepherd's purse tincture.

MENOPAUSE

Menopause can be a difficult transition. The nights sweats, hot flashes, and waves of intense emotions can continue for a few months or last for years.

For night sweats, herbs such as nettle and sage help reduce the sweats, which translates into better sleep. Take the herbs individually as infusions, or in combination. It is up to you.

Chaste tree, ever the woman's ally, can help ease hot flashes when the tincture is taken daily. Codonopsis can help with both hot flashes and riding out the intense, emotional waves.

However, my favorite herb for menopausal symptom relief is dong quai *(Angelica sinensis)*. It helps with hot flashes, palpitations, and spotting, and also relieves thinning and drying of the vaginal tissues. This helps prevent those small tears during intercourse that lead to infections. Not only are the infections absolute misery, but you don't want to have to deal with them when the grid is down or in the midst of civil unrest.

Peppermint tea has a refrigerant, cooling effect. So does peppermint essential oil, which makes a nice, cooling mist when a few drops are added to an atomizer bottle with water. Spritzing a little peppermint mist on the face and neck whenever a hot flash comes on provides instant relief.

Another cooling herb that is wonderful for the skin is rose. You can make your own rose hydrosol much more easily than you can distill rose essential oil. Rose hydrosol has a lovely, light rose scent, and is an excellent toner for the face. Spray it on the face and neck, and let the Queen of Flowers cool hot flashes, care for the skin, and instill a sense of peace.

CONCLUSION

We've covered a lot of information in a small space. But this is hardly an exhaustive work and does not begin to cover every possible scenario you may face during a crisis. However, it should provide you with the information you need to make remedies using some common herbs easily found in nature. Be prepared and be well!

APPENDIX

HERBS AT A GLANCE

The following charts are intended as a quick reference for some of the more common uses of herbs. Use them as a starting point in making your own remedies.

ANALGESICS	
for general pain relief	
HERB	**HOW TO USE HERB**
Arnica	Topically as infused oil, salve, or poultice, especially for arthritis and joint pain. Only use on intact skin.
California poppy	Ingested as tincture for pain.
Cayenne	Topically as infused oil or salve for sore joints and muscles. Dulls the nerves.
Codonopsis	Ingested as tincture or decoction during recovery from injury, migraine, and sore muscles.
Comfrey	Topically as infused oil, salve, or poultice on site of injury.
Echinacea	Topically as tincture or powder on wounds.
Ginger	Topically as infused oil or salve on sore muscles and joints. Ingested as tea, capsules, or in food to reduce overall pain.
Goldenrod	Topically as infused oil or salve for sore joints and muscles.
Lavender	Topically as essential oil, infused oil, or salve directly on site of pain.
Ma huang	Ingested as tincture or decoction during recovery from injury.
Mullein	Topically as infused oil to reduce ear pain, and in salve for arthritic joint relief.

Nettle	Ingested as tisane, tincture, or syrup to reduce swelling and relieve painful joints.
Peppermint	Topically as essential oil or infused oil. Excellent for headache and injuries where cooling is helpful. Do not apply to broken skin.
St. John's wort	Topically as infused oil of the fresh flower. Excellent for nerve pain.
Spilanthes	Topically as tincture directly on tissue. Also known as "toothache plant."
Thyme	Topically as essential oil diluted in a carrier or salve.
Turmeric	Ingested either as powder or fresh rhizome in food. Dehydrated and in capsules.
Usnea	Topically as powder for wounds.
Valerian	Ingested as tincture for pain, especially back and nerve pain.
White willow	Ingested as tincture or decoction for general pain. Use like aspirin.

ANTI-INFLAMMATORY

to soothe red, infected, or injured tissues

HERB	HOW TO USE HERB
Arnica	Topically as infused oil, salve, or poultice applied directly on site of inflammation. Only use on intact skin.
Astragalus	Ingested as tincture or decoction, or in soup stocks.
Berberine	Ingested as tincture for inflammation in the liver or urinary tract. Applied directly as tincture on dental abscesses and oral injuries. Topically as tincture or powder on wounds and skin infections.
Bilberry	Topically as tincture or powder on wounds.
Calendula	Topically as tincture, infused oil, salve, or lotion on skin infections. Added to mouthwashes and rinses for mouth sores and sore throats. Ingested as tisane.
Cayenne	Ingested in food or as tincture, acetum, or capsules to reduce inflammation (tightening) of blood vessels, smooth muscles, and sinus passages. Topically in salve or lotion on sore joints and muscles. Caution: Cayenne can cause inflammation of sensitive tissues. Keep away from the face, eyes, nose, and mouth.
Chinese Skullcap	Ingested as tincture, reduces swelling around the brain due to infection.
Codonopsis	Ingested as tincture, has an anti-inflammatory action on the respiratory system, good for use with wheezing, asthma, and bronchitis.
Cramp Bark	Ingested as tincture, calms inflammation associated with spasms.
Echinacea	Topically in tincture or powder on wounds.
Ginger	Ingested in food or as tisane, juice, acetum, or powdered in capsules. Topically in infused oil and essential oil to make salves and lotions. Great for all types of inflammation from arthritis to food sensitivities to injuries.
Goldenrod	Ingested as tincture, acetum, elixir, or tisane. Topically in infused oil, salve, and lotion. Calms inflammation in the kidneys from urinary tract infections and injuries.

Juniper	Ingested by tincture or topically in an infused oil or salve. Calms inflammation of the kidney, urinary tract, and sore muscles.
Marshmallow	Ingested in syrup or as lozenge for sore throats, and as cold infusion to soothe the mucosa. The cold infusion is an excellent water phase in lotion making.
Mullein	Topically as infused oil from flowers to soothe inflammation from ear infections, arthritis, and skin wounds or infection.
Oats	Topically as oat flour or oatmeal in skin preparations for itchy, dry, red, inflamed skin conditions.
Peppermint	Topically as infused oil, essential oil, or poultice on any itchy, red, inflamed condition. Ingested as tisane. Cooling herb.
Sida	Ingested as tincture, reduces general or localized inflammation from both injury or disease.
Spilanthes	Topically as tincture to numb and reduce inflammation, especially of oral infections and injuries.
Turmeric	Possibly the most potent anti-inflammatory herb available. Ingested in food or capsules to reduce body-wide inflammation. Best consumed with a pinch of black pepper and some fat, such as coconut oil or coconut milk.
Usnea	Topically as powder for wounds.
White willow	Ingested as tincture. Use like aspirin.

ANTISPASMODIC

to stop muscle spasms and relax muscles

HERB	HOW TO USE HERB
American skullcap	Ingested as tincture or tisane to relax muscles that have clenched due to stress or anxiety.
Black cohosh	Ingested as tincture to relieves painful PMS symptoms.
California poppy	Ingested as tincture for painful spasms.
Cayenne	Topically as infused oil or salve and ingested in food or as tincture, acetum, or capsules for muscle spasms.
Cramp bark	Ingested as tincture for PMS symptoms, suspected miscarriage, asthma, and violent coughing.
Ginger	Ingested in food, tisane, juice, or acetum, or as powdered capsules. Ginger is excellent for calming intestinal spasms that occur with food poisoning and intestinal infections. Topically as infused oil and essential oil in salves and lotions.
Lobelia	No better herb for bringing a muscle out of contraction. Ingested as tincture for intensely painful spasms, suspected miscarriage, asthma attacks, and lockjaw. Caution: Low-dose herb; see page 122 for dosing information.
Ma huang	Ingested as tincture or tisane for violent, spastic coughing and asthma attacks.
Motherwort	Ingested as tincture to relieve muscle spasms and PMS symptoms, and to bring muscles out of contraction after being clenched during a stressful event.
Oat tops, Oatstraw	Ingested as tisane, helps to calm spasms caused by nerves or intestinal discomfort.
Peppermint	Ingested as tea to calm intestinal spasms from conditions like Crohn's disease and intestinal infections. Topically to essential oil calm muscle spasms.
Thyme	Inhaled in herbal steams or essential oil in a diffuser to calm bronchial spasms.
Valerian	Ingested as tincture to relax muscles.

ANTIMICROBIAL

for bacterial, viral, fungal, or parasitic infections

HERB	HOW TO USE HERB
Arnica	Bacterial and fungal skin infections.
Berberine	Local bacterial and fungal infections of skin, urinary tract, and intestine.
Burdock	Staphylococcus infections.
Calendula	Fungal infections.
Chinese skullcap	Bacterial, viral, and fungal infections.
Echinacea	Bacterial and viral infections.
Elderberry	Bacterial and viral infections. Mild antibiotic action, highly effective against influenza.
Elecampane	Bacterial, viral, and fungal respiratory infections.
Garlic	Bacterial infections.
Ginger	Bacterial and viral infections. Effective on most strains of the common cold.
Honey	Bacterial infections. Applied topically.
Juniper	Bacterial and viral infections. Effective for respiratory, kidney, and urinary tract infections.
Lavender	Bacterial, viral, and fungal infections.
Lemon balm	Viral infections including herpes outbreaks and respiratory infections.
Licorice	Viral infections. Highly antiviral herb effective for influenza, chickenpox, measles, West Nile virus, and SARS.
Sage	Bacterial and fungal infections.
Sida	Bacterial, viral, fungal, amoebic, and protozoal infections. Systemic antibiotic travels through the blood stream, making it one of a few herbs that might help in cases of sepsis.
Spilanthes	Bacterial infections of the mouth, and spirochete (Lyme) infections.
Thyme	Bacterial, viral, and fungal infections.
Usnea	Bacterial, viral, fungal, and protozoal infections.

DIAPHORETIC

for detoxing through perspiration, cooling body temperature

HERB	HOW TO USE HERB
Calendula	Ingested as tincture.
Elecampagne	Ingested as tincture or tisane.
Garlic	Ingested raw or fermented, or in tincture or acetum.
Ginger	Ingested in tisane or juice.
Goldenrod	Ingested in tisane, tincture, acetum, or elixir.
Hyssop	Ingested in tisane, tincture, or syrup.
Lavender	Ingested in tisane.
Lemon balm	Ingested in tisane, tincture, or glycerite.
Motherwort	Ingested in tisane, tincture, or syrup.
Peppermint	Ingested in tisane, tincture, glycerite, or syrup.
Yarrow	Ingested in tisane or tincture.

ESSENTIAL OILS AT A GLANCE

1% dilution = 6 drops per 1 ounce of carrier oil/finished product

ESSENTIAL OIL	USES
Cedarwood	Use at 2% dilution in lotions for pain and inflammation, such as in rheumatoid arthritis. Inhaling the diffused oil helps relieve congestion and respiratory ailments. Adding to shampoo blends cuts down on dandruff.
Chamomile, German or Roman	Use at 2% dilution. Both oils have similar properties: calming, lowering stress, and relaxing muscles and joints. German chamomile is somewhat better at reducing skin inflammation and redness, while Roman chamomile is somewhat better at reducing pain and inflammation.
Cinnamon	Use at 0.1% dilution. This is a "hot" oil that can irritate skin. Can preserve natural lotions and creams, but may interfere with the scent and reasons for creating the lotion or cream. Antibacterial and antifungal; anti-inflammatory to muscles and joints.
Clove	Use at 0.5% dilution. This is a "hot" oil that can irritate skin. Antibacterial and antifungal oil. Best known for stopping toothaches by applying directly to the tooth/gum, but also makes a wonderful, warming remedy for achy joints.
Ginger	Use at 2% to 5% dilution to produce a warming sensation on skin. Use in steam or bath to manage nausea and relieve cold and flu symptoms.
Helichrysum	Use at 10% dilution for treatment of any injury where skin is intact. Calms inflammation, and reduces pain, discoloration, and swelling from bruising.
Juniper	Use at 0.5% dilution. Add to salves and lotions for pain relief. Can be used as a steam or with a nebulizing diffuser (best option) for respiratory infections. Overuse and extremely high concentrations can irritate the kidneys.
Lavender	Can be used undiluted on most skin areas, but be aware not everyone's skin will react the same way. Useful for headaches, earaches, minor burns, sunburn, bug bites, itching, muscle tension, stress, and congestion. Do not use on deep wounds. It can heal from the outside in, which is not helpful. For formulations, use at 2% dilution. Used to scent laundry, soap, salves, and lotions. Can be used in cleaning products to help disinfect surfaces. For cleaning products and air fresheners, use between 2% to 5%, depending upon how strongly scented you like your products. Blend with tea tree oil for better disinfection.

Lemon	Use at 2% dilution. Uplifting and energizing scent improves mood. Immune stimulant. Excellent for cleaning: Add to soaps or in a 50/50 mix of water and vinegar for an all-purpose surface cleaner and degreaser.
Myrrh	Use at 2% to 5% dilution. Apply to broken skin in the same way that helichrysum is used on intact skin.
Peppermint	Use at 2.5% dilution. Can be used for pain relief due to the high concentration of menthol. Use for migraines, fatigue, nausea, sore muscles, congestion, sunburn, and to cool off someone who is overheating. Can be added to salves, lotions, creams, and soap. In a diffuser, it is a powerful decongestant. Applied in undiluted drops to the temples, it can stop a migraine in its tracks. If undiluted peppermint is too strong, use lavender instead. The oil can be used diluted at 2.5% to 5% in a spray to disinfect surfaces, freshen up a sick room, and repel pests, especially mice and ants.
Sage	Use at 0.5% dilution for cold and flu relief, coughing, and making deodorant.
Tea tree	Use at 2.5% dilution for proven antibacterial, antiviral, and antifungal action. Can often be used undiluted, but some skin may be too sensitive. Always spot-test first. Diluted, it can be used to treat bug bites and itchiness, and added to wound washes to prevent and treat infections. Tea tree oil can be used for puncture wounds to promote healing from the inside out.
Thyme	Use at 1% dilution. Can be added to healing salves and used to prevent infection in cuts and scrapes. It can cause great irritation to the skin, especially sensitive skin. Restrict inhalation time of children in herbal baths or steams.

EXPECTORANT
to make coughing more productive

HERB	HOW TO USE HERB
Chinese skullcap	Ingested as tincture. Important respiratory herb for antibiotic-resistant infections.
Codonopsis	Ingested as tincture. Mild expectorant good as "maintenance" herb for chronic complaints like asthma and chronic bronchitis. Better for preventing attacks than for acute attacks.
Comfrey	Ingested as tisane, for rough coughs, like those associated with whooping cough.
Elecampagne	Ingested as tincture, decoction, or pastilles for relief from deep coughs.
Garlic	Ingested raw, tinctured, fermented, or in syrup. Important herb for respiratory ailments that are very "wet." Not advised for dry coughs.
Goldenrod	Ingested as tincture, tisane, acetum, or elixir to make coughs easier and more productive.
Grindelia	Ingested as tincture for all severe coughing such as in asthma, whooping cough, emphysema, and bronchitis.
Hyssop	Ingested as tincture, tisane, or syrup for all respiratory complaints with a tight chest and difficulty in moving phlegm.
Licorice	Ingested as tisane, lozenge, or syrup to lubricate the mucosa and make coughing easier.
Lobelia	Ingested as tincture for any violent, "thick," or "rough" coughing episode. Caution: Low-dose herb; see page 122 for dosing information.
Ma huang	Ingested as tincture or tisane to make coughing more productive.
Marshmallow	Ingested as cold infusion to moisten the mucosa. Makes coughs more productive by moistening dry coughs and producing more thin mucus to expel.
Mullein	Ingested as tisane, helps ease coughing from all manner of coughs, emollient and soothing to pectoral complaints.
St. John's wort	Ingested as tisane or tincture, take for all serious coughs, including tuberculosis.
Sida	Ingested as a tisane, lubricates mucus membranes, excellent for dry and unproductive coughs.
Thyme	Ingested as tincture, tisane, syrup, or infused honey, or inhaled as herbal steam to thin out mucus from a respiratory infection.

HYPOTENSIVE   VASODILATOR
to lower blood pressure   *to expand blood vessels*

HERB	HOW TO USE HERB
American skullcap	Hypotensive. Ingested as tincture. Especially helpful in lowering blood pressure caused by stress or anxiety.
Astragalus	Hypotensive. Ingested as tincture or tisane, or in soup stock.
Cayenne	Vasodilator. Ingested as tincture or acetum, or powdered in food or capsules. Fast acting.
Cleavers	Hypotensive. Ingested as tincture, tisane, or juice.
Codonopsis	Hypotensive. Ingested as tincture.
Garlic	Hypotensive and vasodilator. Ingested raw or fermented, or as tincture or acetum.
Ginger	Hypotensive and vasodilator. Ingested in food or as tisane, tincture, or juice.
Hawthorn	Hypotensive. Ingested as tisane or tincture.
Lavender	Hypotensive. Ingested as tisane.
Nettle	Hypotensive. Ingested as tisane of the leaves or tincture of the seeds. Helpful in cases where kidney distress is causing hypertension.

NERVINE   ANXIOLYTIC   SEDATIVE
soothes nerves   *anti-anxiety*   *sleep-inducing*

Herb	How to Use Herb
American skullcap	Nervine and mildly sedative. Ingested as tincture to calm someone under great stress. Helpful in fighting insomnia from stress and tension.
California poppy	Anxiolytic and sedative. Ingested as tincture or tisane. Potent muscle relaxant, helps sedate someone even when in pain (if dose is strong enough). Combines well with many mood-enhancing and sedative herbs.
Chinese skullcap	Nervine and mildly sedative. Ingested as tincture.
Cramp bark	Nervine. Ingested as tincture to relieve anxiety.
Grindelia	Sedative, some may find it relaxing while in others it may induce sleep. Ingested as tincture.
Lavender	Nervine and mildly sedative. Ingested as tisane, inhaled as herbal steam or essential oil, or topically as essential oil or infused oil to create a sense of peace and calm.
Lemon balm	Nervine, anxiolytic, and sedative. Ingested as tincture or tisane. Safe herb for calming children or pregnant women. Children and pregnant women may prefer glycerite to tincture.
Motherwort	Nervine and anxiolytic. Ingested as tincture for feeling safe, secure, and nurtured.
Mullein	Nervine and sedative, good for helping a person with violent coughing get some needed rest.
Oats	Nervine. Ingested as tisane of oat straw of milky oat tops. Mildly sedative, calming, nurturing sensation.
St. John's wort	Nervine and anxiolytic. Ingested as tincture or powdered in capsules. Renowned for ability to relieve depression.
Valerian	Nervine, anxiolytic, and sedative. Ingested as tincture or decoction. Promotes deep relaxation, especially ability to sleep with pain.

VULNERARY

assists wound healing

HERB	HOW TO USE HERB
Arnica	Topically as tincture on unbroken skin where there is deep bruising from blunt force.
Berberine	Topically as tincture powder on wounds.
Calendula	Topically as tincture to speed healing of skin conditions, especially sunburns.
Comfrey	Topically as infused oil or poultice for surface tissue healing and bruising only. Heals too fast for deep wounds, which must heal from the inside out. Comfrey may heal the top layers too quickly, leaving the inside vulnerable to infection. Ingestion as tisane to help bones heal after break and internal injuries.
Echinacea	Topically as tincture or powder on wounds.
Garlic	Ingested raw, tinctured, fermented, or in syrup to stimulate immune response and speed healing of wounds.
Lavender	Topically as essential oil or infused oil to heal wounds.
Plantain	Topically as poultice or salve to speed wound healing. Effective for burns, bites, cuts, and scrapes.
St. John's wort	Topically as infused oil combined with honey. Makes an ideal deep wound healing remedy that heals from the inside out.
Yarrow	Topically as tincture or poultice to control blood. Can stop internal bleeding as well as bleeding in deep wounds.

GLOSSARY: ACTIONS OF HERBS

Actions are what an herb does. They describe the impact of the herb on the body. The term "herb" is used very loosely, as is common practice among herbalists, to refer not only to plants but also fungi, lichens, and other natural substances.

It is important to know what actions an herb has, so that you can choose an effective as well as safe herb. For example, an herb that acts as a blood thinner is not appropriate for someone taking a prescription blood thinner. Likewise, it is not appropriate to give a sedative herb to someone getting behind the wheel of a car.

Here is a list of actions and an explanation of what each means. Use it in conjunction with Chapter 4, Materia Medica.

Anti-allergenic: Reduces allergic response to allergens.

Adaptogenic: Encourages homeostasis (equilibrium) and improves response to stress. The effect may be stimulating or calming, depending on the imbalance to be righted.

Antiarrhythmic: Stabilizes irregular heart rhythms.

Agonist: Substance that binds to a receptor site, resulting in a physiological response, either increasing or decreasing the cell's activity.

Analgesic: Reduces pain.

Antibacterial: Effective against bacteria.

Anti-cancer: May reduce the incidence of cancer, may inhibit certain types of cancer cells from proliferating, and may inhibit some risk factor of cancer.

Antidiabetic: Reduces diabetic symptoms and helps maintain healthy blood sugar levels.

Anti-diarrhea: Relieves diarrhea.

Anti-ecchymotic: Reduces bruising.

Anti-emetic: Effective against nausea and vomiting.

Anti-fungal: Effective against fungi.

Anti-inflammatory: Reduces inflammation.

Antimalarial: Fights malaria.

Antimicrobial: Destroys or inhibits the growth of microorganisms, such as bacteria, viruses, fungi, and protozoa.

Antioxidant: Inhibits cellular oxidation and damage from oxidative stress by controlling or eliminating free radicals.

Antiparasitic: Kills parasites.

Antiperspirant: Reduces perspiration (sweat).

Antiprotozoal: Kills protozoa.

Antipruritic: Relieves itching.

Antipyretic: Lowers fever; febrifuge.

Antirheumatic: Relieves symptoms of rheumatism.

Antiseptic: Prevents the growth or action of micro-organisms.

Antispasmodic: Relaxes and interrupts muscle spasms and muscle cramping.

Antisteatosis: Reduces liver fat.

Antitussive: Relieves cough.

Anti-venom: In the medical world, a serum containing the specific antibodies to fight the venom of snakes, spiders, and scorpions. For our purposes, an anti-venom is any herb or natural substance that helps the body fight off such venom.

Antiviral: Effective against viruses.

Anxiolytic: Calms anxiety.

Astringent: Causes a tightening of tissues and mucosa, resulting in a protective barrier.

Bitter/Bitter tonic: Stimulates the digestive process through the taste of "bitter" and contact with gastrointestinal tissue, stimulates upper gastrointestinal tract functions. Also stimulates appetite, general health, and immune function.

Cardioprotective: Protects the heart.

Cardiotonic: Imparts a tonic effect to the heart.

Carminative: Prevents and/or relieves the formation of gas in the gastrointestinal tract.

Cell proliferator: Encourages tissue growth through multiplication of new cells.

Cholagogue: Promotes the discharge of bile down and out of the system, through the intestines, by contraction of the gall bladder.

Choleretic: Stimulates bile production in the liver.

Decongestant: Relieves and clears sinus and upper respiratory congestion.

Demulcent: Relieves irritation by moistening mucus membranes, resulting in a moist, protective coating of the membranes.

Depurative: Promotes detoxification by eliminating metabolic wastes from the body. Formerly referred to as "blood purifier."

Depurative: Aids in detoxification and elimination of metabolic waste.

Diaphoretic: Induces sweating.

Diuretic: Stimulates the elimination of fluid from temporary edema.

Emetic: Causes vomiting.

Emmenagogue: Brings on a delayed menses. This is not the same as an abortifacient (drug or other substance causing an abortion). Out of an abundance of caution, I recommend avoiding the use of emmenagogues during pregnancy.

Emollient: Soothes, softens, and moisturizes skin.

Estrogenic: Causing an effect similar to the activity of an estrogen without actually being/containing an estrogen.

Expectorant: Promotes drainage and thinning of mucus to make coughing more productive and comfortable.

Febrifuge: Reduces fever; antipyretic.

Galactagogue: Increases milk production.

Hematoprotectant: Protects the blood.

Hepatoprotective: Protects the liver.

Hormone modulating: Modulates and balances a hormone's production.

Hypoglycemic: Lowers blood glucose.

Hypolipidemic: Lowers lipids in the blood.

Hypotensive: Lowers blood pressure.

Immunomodulator: Modulates and balances immune response.

Immunostimulant: Stimulates immune response.

Immunotonic: Supports and strengthens the immune system and its ability to respond, but is not a trigger to immune response like an immunostimulant would be.

Laxative: Encourages bowel movements.

Mucous membrane trophorestorative: Strengthens the integrity of the mucous membranes and helps restore the intestinal and respiratory mucosa.

Nephroprotective: Protects the kidneys.

Nervine: Impacts the nerves and/or nervous system. May calm or stimulate the autonomic nervous system, which controls the fight-or-flight response.

Neuroprotective: Protects neurons from injury or degradation.

Peripheral circulatory stimulant: Increases circulation to the extremities.

Radioprotective: Protects against radiation.

Refrigerant: May reduce body temperature or create a cooling sensation on the skin.

Rubefacient: Stimulates circulation.

Sedative: Induces a state of deep relaxation, calms a person in distress, and may cause drowsiness. Sedatives can be sleep-inducing, but not all people will react as strongly.

Spasmolytic: Reduces muscle spasms.

Stimulant: Temporarily increases activity, process, or efficiency of an organ, system, or organism.

Styptic: Stops bleeding.

Synergistic: Causes the potency of every herb in the formula to increase.

Tonic: Restores, invigorates, and strengthens an organ or system.

Trophorestorative: A substance safe for long-term use that provides nourishment and replenishment at a deep level so that restoration of function is possible. Capable of restoring health and function to an organ or system from near failure.

Vasodilator: Relaxes and widens the smooth muscle cells of the blood vessels. This action reduces blood pressure.

Vasoprotective: Protects the integrity of blood vessels, especially the small capillaries that diffuse oxygen into tissue.

Vermifuge: Destroys and/or expels parasitic worms.

Vulnerary: Heals wounds.

RESOURCES

For more information on herbal medicine, visit my website, www
.HerbalPrepper.com, for articles, podcasts, a membership program, and
online herbal education.

RECOMMENDED READING

Aromatherapy

Aromatherapy for Health Professionals, 4th edition by Shirley Price and
Len Price. London: Churchill Livingstone, 2011.

The Aromatherapy Book: Applications and Inhalations by Jeanne Rose.
Berkeley, CA: North Atlantic Books, 1993.

The Directory of Essential Oils: Includes More Than 80 Essential Oils by
Wanda Sellar. London: Random House UK, 2005.

Essential Oil Safety: A Guide for Health Care Professionals, 2nd edition by
Robert Tisserand and Rodney Young. London: Churchill Livingstone,
2014.

Herbal Books

The Book of Herbal Wisdom: Using Plants as Medicines by Matthew Wood.
Berkeley, CA: North Atlantic Books, 1997.

*Herbal Antibiotics: Natural Alternatives for Treating Drug-Resistant
Bacteria,* 2nd edition by Stephen Harrod Buhner. North Adams, MA:
Storey Publishing, 2012.

*Herbal Antivirals: Natural Remedies for Emerging and Resistant Viral
Infections* by Stephen Harrod Buhner. North Adams, MA: Storey
Publishing, 2013.

Herbal Healing for Women: Simple Home Remedies for Women of All Ages by Rosemary Gladstar. New York: Simon & Schuster, 1993.

Herbal Materia Medica by Michael Moore. Bisbee, AZ: Southwest School of Botanical Medicine, 1995. (Available as a downloadable PDF from http://www.swsbm.com/ManualsMM/MatMed5.pdf)

The Herbal Medicine-Maker's Handbook: A Home Manual by James Green. New York: Crossing Press, 2000.

Medical Herbalism: The Science and Practice of Herbal Medicine by David Hoffman. Rochester, VT: Healing Arts Press, 2003.

Nutritional Herbology: A Reference Guide to Herbs by Mark Pedersen. Warsaw, IN: Whitman Publications, 2015.

The Practice of Traditional Western Herbalism: Basic Doctrine, Energetics, and Classification by Matthew Wood. Berkeley, CA: North Atlantic Books, 2004.

Principals and Practice of Phytotherapy: Modern Herbal Medicine, 2nd edition by Kerry Bone and Simon Mills. London: Churchill Livingstone, 2013.

Holistic Health

Holistic Anatomy: An Integrative Guide to the Human Body by Pip Waller. Berkeley, CA: North Atlantic Books, 2010.

Medical Preparedness/First Aid

Living Ready Pocket Manual—First Aid: Fundamentals for Survival by James Hubbard. Blue Ash, OH: F + W Media, 2013.

The Survival Medicine Handbook: A Guide for When Help Is Not on the Way by Joseph Alton and Amy Alton. Weston, FL: Doom and Bloom, 2013.

Midwifery and Women's Health

Birth Emergency Skills Training: Manual for Out-of-Hospital Midwives by Bonnie Gruenberg. Duncannon, PA: Birth Muse Press, 2008.

A Book for Midwives: Care for Pregnancy, Birth, and Women's Health by Susan Klein, Suellen Millar, and Fiona Thomson. Berkeley, CA: Hesperian Foundation, 2013.

Heart and Hands: A Midwife's Guide to Pregnancy and Birth by Elizabeth Davis. Berkeley, CA: Celestial Arts, 2004.

Holistic Midwifery: A Comprehensive Textbook for Midwives in Homebirth Practice, Vol. 1: Care During Pregnancy by Anne Frye. Portland, OR: Labrys Press, 2010.

Taking Charge of Your Fertility: The Definitive Guide to Natural Birth Control, Pregnancy Achievement, and Reproductive Health by Toni Weschler. New York: William Morrow Paperbacks, 2006.

Nutrition and Fermented Foods

Nourishing Traditions: The Cookbook that Challenges Politically Correct Nutrition and the Diet Dictocrats by Sally Fallon and Mary Enig. Washington, DC: NewTrends Publishing, Inc., 2003.

Nutritional Herbology: A Reference Guide to Herbs by Mark Pedersen. Warsaw, IN: Whitman Publications, 2015.

Wild Fermentation: The Flavor, Nutrition, and Craft of Live-Culture Foods by Sandor Ellix Katz and Sally Fallon. White River Junction, VT: Chelsea Green Publishing, 2003.

Soap Making

The Everything Soapmaking Book: Learn How to Make Soap at Home with Recipes, Techniques, and Step-by-Step Instructions by Alicia Grosso. Avon, MA: Adams Media, 2013.

Soap Crafting: Step-by-Step Techniques for Making 31 Unique Cold-Process Soaps by Anna-Marie Faiola. North Adams, MA: Storey Publishing, 2013.

The Soapmaker's Companion: A Comprehensive Guide with Recipes, Techniques, and Know-How by Susan Miller Cavitch. North Adams, MA: Storey Publishing, 1997.

WEBSITES

Education/Research

Doom and Bloom Survival Medicine, http://www.doomandbloom.net

Henriette's Herbal Homepage, http://www.henriettes-herb.com

Herbal Medicine and EarthSpirit Teachings, Herbalist, http://www.robinrosebennett.com

Herbal Prepper, http://www.herbalprepper.com

The Human Path, http://www.thehumanpath.org

The Medicine Woman's Roots, http://www.bearmedicineherbals.com

A Modern Herbal by Mrs. M. Grieve, http://www.botanical.com

Prepper Broadcasting Network, http://www.prepperbroadcasting.com

PubMed, http://www.ncbi.nlm.nih.gov/pubmed

Sage Mountain Herbal Education Center, http://www.sagemountain.com

Southwest School of Botanical Medicine, http://www.swsbm.com

The Survival Doctor, http://www.thesurvivaldoctor.com

Publications

The Essential Herbal Magazine, http://www.essentialherbal.com

Plant Healer Magazine, http://www.planthealermagazine.com

Prepare Magazine, http://www.preparemag.com

Organizations

American Herbalists Guild, http://www.americanherbalistsguild.com

Free Fire Cider, http://www.freefirecider.com

Handcrafted Soap and Cosmetic Guild, http://www.soapguild.org

National Association for Holistic Aromatherapy, https://www.naha.org

National Health Freedom Coalition, http://www.nationalhealth
freedom.org

Seeds

Horizon Herbs, https://www.horizonherbs.com

My Patriot Supply, http://www.mypatriotsupply.com

Sand Mountain Herbs, http://www.sandmountainherbs.com

Suppliers

Alchemical Solutions, http://www.organicalcohol.com

Bulk Herb Store, http://www.bulkherbstore.com

Cultures for Health, http://www.culturesforhealth.com

Jean's Greens, http://www.jeansgreens.com

Mountain Rose Herbs, https://www.mountainroseherbs.com

SKS Bottle and Packaging, http://www.sks-bottle.com

Soaper's Choice, http://www.soaperschoice.com

Wilderness First Aid Courses

The Human Path, http://www.thehumanpath.org

National Outdoor Leadership School, http://www.nols.edu

GENERAL INDEX

Note: Page numbers in **bold** indicate materia medica properties, preparation, and precautions summaries.

A

Accessibility, of natural medicine, 5

Aceta (acetum), 12, 34–35, 51. *See also* Oxymels

Activated charcoal, 17, 25, 138, 152–153, 154

Ailments. *See Index of Ailments*

Alcohol, 9–11
  avoiding, alternatives for, 51
  disinfecting with, 10–11
  grain, 11
  homemade, legal considerations, 10
  ingestion precaution, 11, 33
  isopropyl (ISO), 11
  percent of, 32–34, 50–51
  properties and uses, 9–11
  storing/shelf life, 10
  for tinctures, 9–11, 32–34, 35–36, 50–51
  types and strengths, 10
  vinegar as alternative for, 11, 12
  vodka, brandy, wine, 11

American skullcap, **53–54**, 158, 202, 208, 209

Analgesics (general pain relief), 198–199. *See also specific analgesics*

Anti-Allergy Tea, 182

Anti-anxiety herbs. *See* Anxiolytics

Anti-Infection Salve, 125–126

Anti-Inflammatory Capsules, 126–127

Anti-inflammatory herbs, 200–201. *See also specific herbs*

Anti-Parasitic/Protozoan Tincture, 127

Anti-Scar Salve, 128

Antibacterial Tincture, 128–129

Antibiotics. *See* Antimicrobial herbs

Antifungal Baby Balm, 185

Antimicrobial herbs, 203. *See also specific herbs*

Antispasmodic herbs, 202. *See also specific herbs*

Antiviral Tincture, 129–130

Anxiolytics, 209. *See also specific anxiolytics*

Apple cider vinegar, making, 12

Arnica, 44, **54–55**, 146–147, 156, 157, 179, 198, 200, 203, 210

Aspirin alternative. *See* White willow

Astragalus, **55**, 168, 200, 208

Ayurveda, 3, 177–178

B

Bartering, natural medicine and, 6

Beeswax, 40
  lotions with, 48
  properties and uses, 14
  salves with. *See* Salves, specific
  scale for measuring, 25

Bennett, Robin Rose, 190

Bentonite clay, 16–17, 152–153, 154

Berberine
  Anti-Parasitic/Protozoan Tincture with, 127–128
  for candida/insulin resistance, 172
  Dental Infection Tincture and Mouthwash with, 135–136
  for diabetes care, 178
  Eye Infection Wash/Compress with, 140–141
  properties and uses, **56–58**, 200, 203, 210
  for salmonella, 137
  Sore Throat Spray with, 155
  urinary tract infection tincture with, 159
  Wound Care Tincture with, 160–161
  Wound Wash with, 161–162

Bilberry, **58–59**, 159, 200

Birch bark tea, 179

Birth control, 189–191

Dong quai, 129, 181, 195
Dosages
    for children, 122
    for elderly, 123
    guidelines, 51, 122–123
    for overweight adults, 122–123
    for pregnant and nursing women, 122
Drying herbs, 9, 101

E

Ear Infection Drops, 138–139
Earache Remedy, 139–140
Ease of use, 5
Echinacea
    Antibacterial Tincture with, 128–129
    Antiviral Tincture with, 129–130
    for colds/flu, 56, 83, 182–183
    Dental Infection Tincture and
        Mouthwash with, 135
    for E. coli, 138
    ear drops with, 139
    Elderberry and Echinacea Elixir, 183
    Eye Infection Wash/Compress with,
        140–141
    properties and uses, **74–76**, 102, 198,
        200, 210
    snake-bite tincture with, 153
    Sore Throat Spray with, 155
    Wound Care Tincture with, 160–161
Effectiveness, of natural medicine, 5
Elder (elderberry), 38–39, **76–77**, 129,
    182, 183–184, 203
Elderberry and Echinacea Elixir, 183
Elderly, dosage considerations for, 123
Elecampane, **78**, 203
Electuaries, 42
Elixirs, 39–40
    for common cold/flu, 182–183
    Elderberry and Echinacea Elixir, 183
    goldenrod, 84, 200, 204
    syrups vs., 39
    uses for, 39–40
Emulsifiers, 47–48
Equipment, 25–26
Essential oils, 18–24, 205–206
    blending, 22
    carrier oils for, 20
    concentration levels, 20
    considerations for stocking, 19–20
    containers for, 24

contraindications, 24
distillation of, 18, 20
getting advice on, 23
at a glance, 205–206
GRAS status, 23
growing plant materials for, 18
hype behind, 22–24
labels for, 26, 121
properties and uses, 18–21, 22–24
safely using, 23–24
storing/shelf life, 19
tinctures and, 19–20
Everyday care
    ailments and aids. *See Index of Ailments*
    overview of, 163–164
Expectorants, 207. *See also specific herbs*
Eye Infection Wash/Compress, 140–141

F

Fenugreek, 178
Fermented foods. *See* Lacto-fermentation
    (fermented foods)
Fertility Awareness Method (FAM),
    189–190
Fire cider, 165, 167–169, 170, 176
First aid, administering, 120–121
First aid kit. *See also Index of Ailments*
    administering first aid and, 120–121
    containers for, 121
    dosage considerations, 122–123
    herbs in, 121
    individual vs. combined infusions, 127
    labeling remedies, 121
    needs assumptions, 119–120
Fitness tonic, 173–174
Food
    chronic illness and malnutrition,
        170–171
    as medicine, and medicine as, 38, 163
    sugar and sickness, 169
Fracture and Broken Bones Poultice, 141
French press, 28, 179
Funnels, 26

G

Garlic
    Anti-Parasitic/Protozoan Tincture
        with, 127
    Antibacterial Tincture with, 128–129
    boosting immune system, 167–168

Vinegar, 11–13
  as alcohol alternative, 11, 12
  disinfecting with, 12–13
  making, 12
  properties and uses, 11–13
  shelf life, 27
  testing strength/pH of, 12
  for tinctures (aceta), 12, 34–35
Vulnerary herbs, 210. *See also specific herbs*

W

Weight
  dosage considerations and, 122–123
  obesity and, 57, 64, 169, *172–174*
White willow, 6–7, **116–117**, 148–149,
  179, 199, 201
Wide-mouth funnels, 26

Wild carrot seeds, 189–191
Willow. *See* White willow
Wines, herbal, 35–36
Women, natural medicine for, 163–164.
  See also Index of Ailments
Wood, Matthew, 3
Wound, Burn, or "SHFT" Honey,
  159–160
Wound Care Tincture, 160–161
Wound Powder: Antibacterial, 161
Wound Wash, 161–162

Y

Yarrow, **118**, 144, 160, 161, 195, 204, 210
Yellow Dock and Molasses Syrup, 193

INDEX OF AILMENTS

Note: Page numbers in *italics* indicate primary references.

ACKNOWLEDGMENTS

Thank you to my entire family: to my husband and my beautiful children, who are the reason I do what I do, and to my father and my in-laws for your support and indulging my demanding and crazy schedule.

Thank you to "Old One Eye" for your inspiration, wisdom, and intervention, even when it was relentless; a gift for a gift.

Many thanks to Chuck Hudson for nudging me into talking to preppers about herbal medicines. Your instigation kick-started events into motion that resulted in this book. I'm proud to count you among my friends.

Much gratitude and thanks to Linda Patterson. Taking your herbal course was life-changing. While it looks very different now, my final project for your class has grown and changed since then, to eventually become this book.

Thank you to Casie Vogel and everyone at Ulysses Press for your support and expertise, without which this book would not have materialized.

Thank you to my readers, listeners, and students, who are some of the most intelligent, curious, caring, and dedicated people I've ever had the pleasure to know. Your support has meant more to me than I can express.

Finally, to the soil, herbs, fungi, lichens, trees, honeybees, and oceans, for your many lessons and gifts. I am, forever, your humble student.

ABOUT THE AUTHOR

Cat Ellis is a practicing herbalist and dedicated prepper. Her love of herbs began in the 1990s when herbs helped her recover from the flu. Cat now has her own practice and teaches herbal medicine. She is also a massage therapist certified in MotherMassage, and belongs to the American Herbalists Guild.

Because of economic uncertainty and a desire for wider freedoms, Cat became interested in survivalism and homesteading in 2008. She describes prepping as having "hundreds of practical hobbies," like gardening, canning, and self-defense.

Cat's love of herbal medicine merged with her love of prepping, resulting in her website www.HerbalPrepper.com. Cat has been published in *Prepare* magazine, and she hosts the show "Herbal Prepper Live" on Prepper Broadcasting.

Cat Ellis lives on the New England coast with her beekeeper husband and homeschools her children.